Ten minutes for the family

Providing holistic health and mental health care is a key challenge facing general practitioners and their teams. Primary care provision has moved from doctor-controlled to patient-centred consultations, with greater emphasis on collaboration. Patients must also be considered within the contexts of their wider families, relationships and health beliefs. There is now a strong evidence base to support the use of systemic approaches in managing many mental health and relationship problems.

Ten Minutes for the Family is a practical guide written by full-time front-line practitioners for health professionals working in primary care who want to improve their skills and effectiveness for working with problem patients and their families. Step-by-step it introduces both the theory and the practice of systemic approaches – from interviewing patients in routine consultations to conducting family crisis meetings. It provides concrete suggestions for using simple family therapy techniques and encourages systematic and constructive thinking about individual cases. Case histories and vignettes are used extensively to illustrate the techniques and key points are highlighted.

Eia Asen is Clinical Director and Consultant Child and Adolescent Psychiatrist at the Marlborough Family Service. He is also a family therapist of international renown. **Dave Tomson** is a GP on Tyneside with a background in family work, education, learning and service development. He has had lecturer posts at local universities and is now a freelance consultant in the development of patient centred primary care. **Venetia Young** is a GP in Penrith, Cumbria and a family therapist at the Psychotherapy department in Carlisle. As GP Mental Health Lead for Eden Valley PCT she is involved in service redesign and mental health training for primary care and community staff. **Peter Tomson** is a retired GP, previously Honorary Senior Lecturer at St Bartholomew's Hospital, a member of one of Michael Balint's original groups and a pioneer of introducing systemic practices into primary care.

Ten minutes for the family

Systemic interventions in primary care

Eia Asen, Dave Tomson,
Venetia Young and Peter Tomson

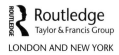

Routledge
Taylor & Francis Group

LONDON AND NEW YORK

First published 2004
by Routledge
11 New Fetter Lane, London EC4P 4EE

Simultaneously published in the USA and Canada
by Routledge
29 West 35th Street, New York, NY 10001

Routledge is an imprint of the Taylor & Francis Group

© 2004 Eia Asen, Dave Tomson, Venetia Young and Peter Tomson

Typeset in Times by
Florence Production Ltd, Stoodleigh, Devon
Printed and bound in Great Britain by
TJ International Ltd, Padstow, Cornwall

British Library Cataloguing in Publication Data
A catalogue record for this book is available from the British Library

Library of Congress Cataloging in Publication Data
A catalog record for this book has been requested

ISBN 0–415–30188–2 (hbk)
ISBN 0–415–30189–0 (pbk)

Contents

INTRODUCTION   vii

1   SYSTEMIC PRACTICE IN A CHANGING WORLD   1

2   INGREDIENTS OF THE SYSTEMIC APPROACH   11

3   THE EVOLUTION OF SYSTEMIC WORK   32

4   QUESTIONING AND REFLECTING ON THE AGENDA   45

5   THE FAMILY WITHIN US – GENOGRAMS   64

6   NOT GOING ROUND IN CIRCLES   78

7   FAMILY TRANSITIONS   90

8   ASSESSING, REFLECTING AND CONNECTING   102

9   WORKING WITH COUPLES   123

10 DANCING WITH THE FAMILY   143

11 THE FAMILY IN CRISIS   160

12 ROOTS, TRUNK, SHOOTS, FRUITS AND SEEDS:
    PUTTING IT ALL TOGETHER   181

    REFERENCES   192

    INDEX   197

Introduction

This introduction covers:
- O Typical primary care scenarios
- O Systemic practice ideas
- O When to use the approach
- O How to use and navigate the book

Scene: a group practice. Monday morning.

Next please . . .

Mrs W, age 36, has made yet another appointment – the sixth in the past three weeks. 'Oh, not her again,' thinks the receptionist, 'what could it be today? We've had dizzy spells, headaches, palpitations, breathlessness and back pain.' Dr J reviews her case notes briefly. Various routine investigations have failed to establish any organic cause, she denies that there are any worries about marriage, money and children. 'Doctor, I have got pains in my chest, especially if I take a deep breath.' Dr J suspects that she is hyperventilating, but nevertheless agrees to listen to her chest. 'Is it serious, doctor?' 'No, I shouldn't think so.' Dr J feels a bit lost and wonders what is going on. He asks his colleague, Dr C, to help him out and see the patient.

MRS W:	*'I don't feel at all well, doctor.'*
DR C:	*'I don't feel I know you very well – just before you go on could you tell me a little more about yourself and your family?'*
MRS W:	*'My husband . . .'*
DR C:	*'So, what does your husband make of it all?'*
MRS W:	*'My husband? Well, he would say that I worry too much about my mother.'*
DR C:	*'If he was here, what would he say – how does he see the problem?'*
MRS W:	*'He knows my mother isn't well, but he thinks I spend too much time with her anyway.'*
DR C:	*'Would he be right thinking that?'*
MRS W:	*'Yes and no . . . it's always been a bit of a problem . . . he has sometimes said that I am married to my mother and not to him. And it's worse now . . . I feel caught . . . it makes me feel dizzy just thinking about it.' [takes a deep breath]*

DR C: *(thinks: 'I think I'm onto something here, perhaps a family approach would work here. I wish I knew how to work with couples and families!') 'Would you like your husband to come here with you?'*

MRS W: *'I don't think he would want to come.'*

Dr C need not panic about having to manage a twosome, or even a threesome, in the consulting room. Usually it is unnecessary to bring in the key players in person. Mrs W can be helped on her own, by using her family as a context within which to think about her symptoms. But what is happening in this consultation? By asking simple questions the picture has been enlarged. Instead of two people in the consulting room, we now have four (patient, doctor, the mother and the husband) – the latter two invisible but nevertheless very present. When we feel 'stuck' in our work with patients we long for another view. It is possible to generate new views simply by asking patients how they think they are being viewed by others. Mrs W is asked to see herself through the eyes of others. This offers her – and the clinician – new perspectives. The physical symptoms come alive as she talks about family dynamics. This will make her think – and maybe act differently. It is the beginning of systemic work.

Systemic work in primary care

Ten minutes for the family seems very ambitious. How is it possible to see a whole family in such short a time and do justice to its complexities? In some ways it can never do full justice, but what is possible is to consistently and creatively take account of context and the family. This can be done in many different ways:

- Simply by thinking differently
- Looking at case notes from a new perspective
- Seeing the patient and their illness from a different angle in a routine consultation
- Looking at the multiple living contexts over subsequent appointments
- Seeing more than one family member
- Having conversations with colleagues to widen the lens.

Working systemically is like having a series of lenses that you can snap onto your camera and alter the perspective of the problem seen. When patients come to the consulting room it is almost as if they are fish plucked out of the water and sitting in the frying pan of the consultation. Sometimes both patient and clinician may struggle to avoid being cooked. This book is about seeing the fish swimming back in their water and discovering how this can be done in 10 minutes or in the occasional double appointment, an approach that respects the time frames and boundaries of primary care.

This book is about understanding and unravelling the systems within which we work and live. It is about the relationships individuals have within these contexts – relationships with each other, with symptoms and diseases and illnesses, with environment, with beliefs and stories. It is about a framework for understanding practice and offers a way of putting these contexts to use, for the patient and for the clinician. It is an interactional, interpersonal rather than intrapersonal approach. It addresses concrete relationships rather than internal objects. Primary care is full of the stories of people and their families.

Next please . . .

Have you, the district nurse, ever noticed how often it appears that elderly couples seem to take it in turns to be ill? Have you ever wondered why or how this often appears to happen, as you, yet again, ask the GP to find a respite bed? Do you wonder whether they are happily married, or whether they are managing a huge burden of illness that they have to share?

Next please . . .

Two consecutive patients present to you, the GP, in your morning surgery with back pain. The first, Mr S, age 78, put his back out shifting a bag of sand for his grandson. He already has bad arthritis and appears simply to want confirmation that his spondylitis has been exacerbated. He doesn't like pain killers and is soon leaving again with a smile and an 'I expect it will get better in a few days' as he goes. The next patient, Mr P, is 36 and has put his back out picking up a tube of toothpaste from the bathroom floor. He brings his partner and is hyper-ventilating as he collapses into a chair. His partner hovers over him with a very worried look on her face. You glance down and note that he saw the nurse practitioner only two weeks ago with a shoulder pain. There is an odd feeling in your body. If you had time to reflect you might identify it as irritation, even dislike. There is simply not time to reflect on where that feeling comes from. But you might wonder why seemingly similar problems present so differ-ently when located in different people's lives.

Next please . . .

You, the nurse practitioner, sit down to a late coffee. Most of the team have left and you have only the practice manager to moan to. Your entire clinic seems to have consisted of either taking blood pressures or smears and seeing patients who seem to invent reasons for coming to see you every week. The practice manager jokes that 'Perhaps they all love you too much'. You shudder at the thought of Mr M being in love with you. As you head out of the common room and back to the treatment room for the next instalment of life's rich tapestry, you muse on the pleasures and dangers of having patients love you and wonder vaguely about depen-dency and then fleetingly as you start again – you wonder about whose dependency is whose.

Next please . . .

You, the practice nurse, have been asked to do an extra post-heart attack visit to Mr R. He remains depressed and lacking in any motivation although, as far as you and the GP can tell, he is quite fit enough to return to work. It is only when you begin to explore with his wife her fears and beliefs about the cause of his heart attack, that it begins to make sense.

Next please . . .

Mrs B brings her 3-year-old son in with a cold and headaches. 'He was burning up last night and crying with it and you know how I worry.' You do and she does. Her elder child very nearly died four years ago after a delayed diagnosis of meningitis – thankfully at a different practice. You, the GP, conduct a thorough history and examination and tell Mrs B that it is just a cold, remind her of what to look out for and see her leave grateful as ever for the reas-surance. It feels nice to be able to do that but right at the back of your mind you wonder when she will become less anxious and what effect it might be having on Charles, the little boy. You wonder if there are ways you can behave differently that might have an effect on the situation – how could she reassure herself?

Next please . . .

Someone you used to see almost weekly before you went on sabbatical appears to have disappeared on your return. You send round an internal e-mail and find out that he is still on the books but has only consulted twice in the last year and was doing well. You announce that you will be taking a sabbatical every year now, and then wonder how you could take a metaphorical sabbatical with several other patients.

Next please . . .

Today you seem to be consulting very poorly. You are irritable and just want the patients out of the surgery. You suddenly find yourself wondering why your husband never, ever, ever organises the family holiday and whether you can fit in a visit to your poorly mum before you pick up the kids from after-school club. You shove these thoughts to the back of your mind as you press the bell for the next patient.

Next please . . .

For the last four weeks you, the health visitor, have been trying to do a sleep programme with Ms W and her 18-month-old son Jack. As you walk into the house this time you are introduced to Ms W's mother, who was on the point of leaving. You persuade her to stay and discover that she and her mother have opposing views about how children should be brought up. Ms W has mentioned this, but it is not until you get them both in the room together that it becomes clear how easily the plans for sleep programmes are being subverted.

Next please . . .

Why on earth does Mrs A, who seems to make your heart sink so badly whenever you see her, seem to get on fine with the new registrar?

Next please . . .

Mr L suffers from recurrent aches and pains in multiple locations. His wife is initially quite worried, but with time she gets increasingly tired of hearing about his constant complaints. She becomes more 'deaf' and less tolerant which Mr L sees as evidence that she simply doesn't care. When he says this, his wife feels accused and becomes more irritable. The children take sides with their father and this results in Mrs L feeling misunderstood. She gets depressed. This, in turn, makes their three pre-adolescent children feel sorry for their mother. Soon they feel torn as to who they should help most. Their school performance suffers. The situation is further compounded by 'well-meaning' interventions from one of the grandmothers. As she gets more and more involved, it now seems to be grandpa's turn to feel left out. He goes and consults his doctor about some stomach problems.

If any of these little vignettes made you wince or laugh or smile ruefully, if you recognised anything of your own experience in them and are at all interested in thinking more about all this, then this book is for you! It is aimed at people who are interested in people and in working with them on navigating their lives more successfully. It may also say something about how to be a happier, more interested and curious primary care clinician, not just in relation to your patients, but also in relation to your other worlds – the practice team, the primary case team, the appraisal team, the mental health subgroup, even the family from which you come! At its simplest it is a book about the primary care consultation – the nodal point between patient (client, user, person, parent, customer) and clinician (nurse, doctor, health visitor, mental health worker).

Thankfully perhaps, the consultation between patient and clinician is still the bedrock of practice and of care. Modern primary care is increasingly complex, with layers of context that make up this complexity. There are ever increasing external pressures on what must be delivered in the consultation. Furthermore, there is increasing complexity in the teams that exist in primary care. There are new managerial contexts, marked by allegedly new concepts such as continued professional development, clinical governance, performance indicators, patient-centred practice and so on. All these reflect changes in the social and political contexts in which care is delivered. This book will also have useful things to say about these various layers of context and offer ways of travelling through this territory, hopefully with more control and more enjoyment than perhaps you experience now.

What is the central idea?

Every individual is embedded in multiple contexts – physical, historical, family, financial, spiritual, cultural and other relationship contexts. The stuff of understanding individuals and their troubles (illnesses, diseases and difficulties) is the stuff of understanding them within, not separate from, their contexts. The aim of this book is to enable primary care workers to work with problem situations, problem patients and problem families, both individually and jointly. 'Working with the family' means engaging in a collaborative relationship with families over time, with a focus both on the treatment and management of illness as well as on the promotion of health. Change can be brought about by providing seemingly simple interventions to what often seem intractable problems. The approach has preventive aspects, it is a way of making sense by looking at a larger picture – the family and the wider context. It is patient-friendly and involves the whole family and/or other significant relationships, if not in person then at least in spirit. It is *not* an invitation to get immersed in people's psychological states and to become depressed or confused in the process.

Next please ...

A GP trainer is talking with his registrar about a patient the registrar has just seen: Mrs J is a middle-aged woman who presented with chest pain. The registrar had asked the usual questions, but recognised that something was missing. Somehow the consultation had gone round the loop twice. He had told her not to worry but wanted to chat it through with the trainer almost as soon as she had left. He still wasn't sure whether there was something 'real' going on here or not. Was it just anxiety or real chest pain? The trainer raised an eyebrow at the idea that there might be 'unreal' things going on but let it pass for now. He said there were lots of possibilities but it might have something to do with the prostate cancer diagnosed in her husband who the trainer had seen two days ago. The registrar's face brightens – the 'ah ha' moment: 'Now that begins to make sense.' The registrar relaxes. 'But then again I also know that her mother and grandfather both died early of heart attacks.' The registrar looks anxious again. 'But then again I am sure it is that family which has the terrible neighbour problem and the daughter who has just returned home after a failed marriage.' The registrar looks relieved again. 'But then again. . . .'

Most of us will be familiar with the above tale of the GP trainer alternatively impressing and exasperating his pupil with the layers of context he was able to summon up, each of which alters the possible meaning of the symptom. But the idea of thinking about individuals as opposed to systems is very deeply embedded in Western medical and nursing culture. Go back and look at the case vignettes presented earlier in this chapter. All of them are about how much symptoms, illnesses and stories are influenced by past and present relationships and contexts – what we might call the 'system' within which the patient has developed and lives. The stalwart old man who is uncomplaining of his back was brought up by a miner who had 25 years in the pit and a mother who died when he was 20, after a long debilitating illness through which she never complained. The younger man brings a quite different set of relationships and influences to his tale.

Health visitors, district nurses, GPs – we all carry some of this knowledge. Why do we not put that knowledge to better use rather than allowing it to become part of why situations stay stuck: 'Oh you will never succeed with that woman. It's all to do with the death of her son. He drowned some years ago – I don't think she will ever be happy again.'

Who might particularly benefit from this approach?

The family approach is applicable in any consultation with patients or clients. It is particularly useful for the following groups.

Somatically fixated patients

Somatising presents challenges for patients and for clinicians. The somatically fixated patient is preoccupied with their body, consulting the doctor endlessly for physical complaints which seem major to the patient and minor to the clinician (fatigue, joint pains, dizziness, vague abdominal pain), none of which appear to respond to any of the treatments offered. Multiple practice attenders, the 'fat file syndrome', present with non-specific symptoms. They are a time-consuming group of 'heartsink' patients (O'Dowd 1988). Many can be helped by bringing in the family, and the clinician's sinking heart can also be helped by this approach! Moreover, if seen early in their 'careers', preventive action can be taken to avoid the development of future chronic help-seeking patterns.

Multiple attenders

Overutilisation of primary care services by the same patient can prove a big problem to a health centre or practice (Westhead 1985, Katon *et al*. 1990). At times, two or more family members may present simultaneously or successively with similar types of problems. Clinicians will think of such a 'ripple effect' when a series of illnesses occur in close temporal sequence within the same family. Huygen (1978), one of the pioneers of a family approach in primary care, did a great job mapping over time the consulting behaviours of family members, and Dowrick (1992) has produced one of the nicest case studies.

Patients with emotional problems

Patients who consult their doctors because of psychological symptoms often themselves point to the interpersonal dimension of their problems. 'Thinking families' gives patients a new perspective: it helps them to see their problems in context. In this way they can make sense of their predicaments and get some guidance as to how to tackle problems with the help of a spouse, parent or friend.

Children who present as having problems

Some children are repeatedly presented to the primary care team with minor illness or behaviour problems. The family approach is particularly relevant when it comes to working with children and their carers. A child who is repeatedly presented as 'the problem' at the surgery may often be an indicator of family discord. Enuresis, faecal soiling, behavioural difficulties, feeding and eating disorders are common presentations. There are also those families whose children frequently attend for urinary tract infections or diarrhoea and vomiting, and who seem never to learn to manage things from experience.

The family in crisis

The primary care team is likely to be consulted at specific times of crisis: at the birth of a child, when a patient is dying, when someone has attempted suicide or in the midst of some dramatic family break-up. Members of the primary care team may be requested to make a domiciliary visit and suddenly face the whole family. Being comfortable talking with the whole family is a necessary prerequisite for helping families to cope with such crises. It is also a time when some of the most successful family work can be done. A crisis is – as the Chinese would have it – a dangerous opportunity!

Addiction-related problems

Excessive alcohol consumption and addiction to prescribed or illicit drugs are problems whose origins or maintenance are often to be found in the individual's home or family circumstances. Repeated requests for a sick note or antacid on Mondays are familiar warning signs. The family approach acknowledges this and shows that in these cases there is frequently family participation: changing the drinking behaviour is more effective when spouses and parents are involved.

Concordance problems

Arriving at successful treatment plans which are acceptable to, and achievable by, patients is one of the major tasks of the clinician. The fact that 50 per cent of antibiotics in the UK are never 'cashed' and numerous other examples of discrepancy between providers and patients about what happens after a consultation, are all evidence of the difficulties in achieving concordance. Family approaches that pay heed to beliefs, narratives and barriers to change can be very useful in improving the chances of success for both patients and their clinicians.

Health promotion work

A considerable amount of time in primary care settings is spent talking with people about weight reduction, risk factor reduction for hypertension, smoking cessation. There is some evidence that taking a family approach to these behavioural issues can be more helpful than constantly trying to work with the individual (Doherty and Campbell 1988).

Clinicians who are stuck or burnt-out or bored

In any survey of patients' views about what they want from health care professionals, listening and engaging with them is usually top of the list. Yet, day-in day-out this can be a challenge for any professional. The systemic approach, at the very least, offers a new way of staying interested. But it also provides some clues as to why certain people trigger feelings of annoyance, or sadness or perhaps most importantly, impotence in us. Systemic practice offers a way to connect things in new light, offers new refreshing perspectives, and will occasionally help you feel that 'today I really consulted like a champion!' and that can't be bad for anyone!

Primary care teams who have too much conflict or too little, or seem sad or sick or angry or . . .

There is little in these ideas that cannot be directed at the system of the primary care team itself. How often have you wondered why you always behave in a certain way when confronted by the senior partner? Why does the receptionist feel marginalised? How is it that the doctors are not sharing crucial information with the health visitors? We are sometimes aware of the steps in the dance of our close personal relationships – what about the 'dances' with members of our health care team?

How to use this book

Above all else we have been motivated in writing this book by a desire to offer something practical and accessible to hard-working and busy front-line primary care staff. The central thread throughout has been to offer examples of things you can do within your current time frames and contexts. There are numerous case examples. We have tried to offer actual forms of words that you can try and we have covered a large territory with a light touch and in our own idiosyncratic way. We make no apologies for this. It will only be useful to you if our enthusiasm for this way of working and thinking comes over in these pages – and if it infects you!

It is our belief that there are a number of simple and key ingredients to being a good primary care practitioner apart from biomedical knowledge:

- Curiosity and interest in others
- A continued interest and enthusiasm for your work
- The habit of reflection on your work and wider concerns
- And perhaps, an acceptance that change in health care is as inevitable as change in the surrounding culture or, indeed, your own age!

With this in mind, we have tried to offer not just a 'main trunk' of ideas, but also a number of other components that make up the whole knowledge tree:

- The '*Roots*' of this way of working – the sources, key texts and some of the founding ideas, indicated by this logo

- The '*Shoots*' or laterals to the main trunk, which connect with the text but may take you into some other reflections on practice, or other avenues to explore, indicated by

- The '*Fruits*' this approach produces: the take-home skills, the *aide-mémoires*, the forms of words, indicated by

- The '*Seeds*' for change in your practice: suggestions for exercises and tasks that help you grow in skills and confidence, indicated by

The text is liberally scattered with patient stories and case reports, identifiable as '*next please . . .*'.

The main text stands alone and can be read without reference to any of the various knowledge tree boxes. Likewise each knowledge tree box can be read as a separate item. For the impatient reader, if you only read the boxes a different but, we hope, useful story will emerge. However, be warned, you may become so curious that you want to read the rest of the book! Wherever possible we have linked and cross-referenced to ease your navigation of the territory. However, we surely will not have referenced all the authors, thinkers, practitioners and most importantly, patients who have influenced and inspired us. There are many and we are grateful to them all. The identities of our patients have been heavily disguised.

This book has an ancestor: *Family Solutions in Family Practice* (Asen and Tomson 1992) was published more than a decade ago. Its two original authors have now been joined by a younger generation of clinicians working in primary care, to bring it up to date for the new millennium.

The first part of the present book – the Introduction and the two following chapters – set the theoretical framework. They introduce the main ideas, look at the specific contexts in which we are working, and argue for the specific role for this way of working. Chapter 3 covers some of the main roots of the ideas and can be dipped into or referred to at any time – or ignored completely if you don't like the intellectual stuff. Chapters 4–9 offer the main techniques and areas of practice that most clinicians will want and find easy to use. These chapters are about working with individuals or a couple of people. Chapters 10 and 11 extend the thinking to working with the whole family. Chapter 12 looks at the thorny issue of how to make lasting changes in the way you practice. It's all very well to get excited by an idea in a book – quite a different matter to use the idea to change your behaviour with the last patient on a Friday afternoon!

Lastly, this is a book that would like to be in dialogue. Systemic practice is a developing field and you, the readers, will hopefully be experimenting with fertile ideas, adapting them to your own contexts and personal styles. Future editions of this book will be made all the richer for a dialogue with you.

Systemic practice in a changing world

This chapter covers:
- ○ Organising contexts for the team as well as for patients
- ○ Split bodies and minds
- ○ Differences between linear and circular causality
- ○ The changing nature of primary care

We have already explained that each individual is part of, and influenced by, a variety of *organising contexts* – physical, historical, financial, spiritual, cultural, family and relational. This not only applies to patients but also to the clinicians working in primary care settings. There is the context of the team which is affected by ever-changing political and economic priorities. New – or old – ideologies shape these priorities. Then there are the professional and personal beliefs that we all bring to our workplace. The systemic approach lends itself to helping clinicians and primary care teams to view their beliefs and actions in context. In reality, many primary care teams do not feel that they work very well together. Just like families, they may work better at some times than others, they contain members with quite different ideas about how to proceed. They have often grown in size over the years but may still be using rules that worked better for families of the 1950s!

We would love to explore the richness of each and every one of these contexts – but you are busy and practical people who want to 'do things'! So we have picked out a few of the cultural and ideological contexts which seem most important to us. By offering systemic perspectives on these 'organising contexts' we hope to offer some liberation from ossified ways of working. But first a word about a word – context. This term is much used and means so many different things, depending on the contexts within which it is used! The GP may see a patient in the context of general practice. The 10-minute consultation is a common time context used in general practice. There is also a person context: the individual, the couple, the family. Families – and individuals – exist in 'living contexts', whether neighbourhoods, countries or indeed cultures. The word context is derived from a Latin verb meaning 'weaving together', thus implying a dynamic phenomenon rather than the static notion the noun conjures up. In the systemic field we look at actions or interactions, at a word or a phrase, in specific contexts, each of which might give these actions or words new meanings. These different contexts are like temporary frames within which we view what people do or say. Generating new frames is an activity many clinicians see as the meat of their work. It is also known as *reframing*, namely placing the 'facts' of the 'same' interactions in another frame which also fits them, thereby changing its conceptual and emotional meaning completely (Watzlawick *et al.* 1974).

Contexts overlap and intermingle. Like threads in shot silk, each one is different and at different times and from different angles they become more or less visible. They weave together to create the backdrop for our everyday practice.

The culture of the individual

In Western culture the supremacy of the individual over the group, the family or the collective has been a fact of intellectual, organisational and cultural life since long before the infamous remark of a recent British Prime Minister that there was no such thing as 'society' but only 'individuals'. Never has this been more evident than in the development of 'Western' medicine, whose whole approach is based on an examination of the individual as object of positivist scientific scrutiny. Where

Coordinated management of meaning (CMM)

CMM (Pearce and Cronen 1980) views communication and interaction within a hierarchy of contexts. It suggests that communication is a social process of coordinating action and managing structure. Social meanings are hierarchically organised so that one level is the context for the interpretation of others. When looking at families, it is generally possible to distinguish five levels of information exchange. At the 'lowest' level we have (1) speech acts, verbal and non-verbal messages such as 'undermining my self-esteem', 'compliment' or 'promise'. These turn into (2) episodes when they become reciprocal: 'Our usual fight about who has a shower first'. A (3) relationship emerges once two or more persons refer to the terms on how they engage: 'She is the leader, I am the follower'. At a 'higher' level there are (4) life scripts, the person's concept of self: 'I am a pessimist, but I am also a realist'. At yet a higher level we have (5) family myths or cultural patterns that locate human experience in a broader frame, legitimising ways of acting and knowing. They refer to general conceptions of how society, family relationships and individual roles work.

This theoretical model is useful when attempting to make sense or create meaning out of seemingly inexplicable or contradictory communications and interactions. Social meanings are hierarchically organised so that one level is the context for the interpretation of others. Different levels of context can be organised in such a way that each is equally the context for and within the other, with changes in each level affecting the meaning of the other. If one context is regarded as 'higher', then the meaning attributed to a speech act or episode will be 'framed' accordingly. For example, if an individual's highest context is his life script (e.g. 'pessimist and realist'), then all speech acts, episodes and relationships may be guided by this view. Yet, if the highest context is cultural patterns (e.g. 'Allah watches over my life'), then the very same speech acts or episodes assume very different meanings. For clinicians it is therefore important to become curious about the highest context in any given communication.

the gaze of this science and practice has risen above the intracellular, it has rarely risen beyond the individual. Disease and, by default, illness are seen as being individual matters, located in individuals or their body parts. Consulting behaviours within most health care settings have demonstrated that, despite current rhetoric to the contrary, most patients are still seen alone, even if other family members may also be present. And if illnesses are seen to reside in the individual, they also need to be 'fixed' by and in the individual. Individuals are seen as having a specific personality independent of their relationships with others.

Systemic practice acknowledges both individual *and* contextual factors. It is particularly interested in the way individuals behave in relation to each other, it assumes that one person's actions and feelings are connected with those of other persons. Illnesses do not just reside in organs and individuals, they are also relational and contextual. When Mrs S brings her depressed husband to see her GP and he denies that he is feeling low with a smile on his face, she is a contextual thinker when she says: 'It's just typical, he's been absolutely miserable until we came in here – now he's going to make a liar of me.'

A systemic clinician will want to make connections, without just validating one person's view at the expense of the other. This can be done by, for example, inviting the husband's reflections or comments: 'Mr S, what is it that your wife has seen or experienced at home that makes her bring you here and say that you are "absolutely miserable"?'

Here the clinician is interested in how each person came to form their specific views. Inviting the husband to look at himself through the eyes of his wife is a step to joint exploration of what seems to be a problematic issue. This can be followed by: 'Are there times when you might be more or less "miserable", as your wife puts it? What's your explanation for this?'

And, a bit later the systemic clinician will want to elicit Mrs S's views about her husband's views. In this way different and differing views become linked.

Much of what clinicians encounter is linked to multiple contexts – if one wants to find the links. 'Pauline [Health visitor], my baby just won't stop crying.' Which clinician has not examined and then just held a crying baby on a night visit, only to see the baby calm down as it relaxes away from its anxious parent? The child has a temperature and is crying with pain or tiredness or misery. The parents try whatever they can and for many reasons lose confidence that crying babies are not all that abnormal. They enlist the, sometimes conflicting, help of others. New or unfamiliar things are tried with the baby who becomes more distressed. This only goes to 'prove' the seriousness of the problem. Finally the health visitor is consulted. She has seen many ill and unhappy babies before. The parents have some confidence that she will know what is going on and – surprise, surprise – often the 'room temperature' and the 'carer temperature' and ultimately the baby's temperature come down. Generally it seems easier to be sure about where the disease (a cold) is located. It is much more difficult to determine the 'site' of the illness or problem – it tends to be 'between' people! Panic attacks can be located in the individual, but their emergence and manifestation are often contextual: the presence of concerned onlookers almost always makes the job of controlling a panic attack harder.

It may still be difficult to see the disease belonging to a context but it is often easy to see that the problem is far wider than the individual. For example, there is good evidence that many of us carry *Streptococcus* bacteria in the oral cavity, but we do not all have tonsillitis all the time. Stressors of various kinds often seem to precipitate the disease of tonsillitis in the individual. But where is the problem – in the tonsils, in the individual, in the context that generates the stress, in the learned responses to that stress in that particular individual or in the family in which they learned these responses? Systemic clinicians tend to broaden the context and ask the patient, at some stage: 'What would be most useful to talk about today – that your throat is tense or that your life is tense?' Clearly such a challenge requires a bit of preparation, but it can be very effective in shifting the focus and can come as a relief to the patient.

Split bodies and minds

A central feature of Western thought has been to split the Mind from the Body. This split is so embedded culturally that it organises most of our perceptions and many of our practices. The split is manifested in disciplines: we have the field of psychiatry versus the specialty of 'internal' medicine. It is also reflected in service structures: we have national standards for delivering mental health services that are quite separate from those for diabetes or heart disease, despite the fact that feeling sad is a better predictor of death after a heart attack than taking aspirin (Mumford *et al.* 1982)! Is a headache in your mind or in your head or in your skull? Where does the head end and the skull start? It can be heart-breaking just thinking about the knots this intellectual schism has caused! No wonder we sometimes have headaches, as our language, our training and the services we work in all coerce us into sorting people and their symptoms into categories: 'You to a heart specialist; you to a psychiatrist.' But which expert is best placed to look after a broken heart? Much of modern medicine seems to encourage our patients to 'dis-integrate' and present different body and mind parts to different specialists, so that we can apply our 'bitsy' remedies.

Systemic practice goes some way towards the aspiration of *integrated practice*. Integrated practice takes as its core value the inextricable and indivisible link of mind and body, the intrinsic relatedness of the physical and the psychological. The playing out of this core value occurs at the level of thinking, of language, of communication, of structure and of organisation. Recipients and providers of care, patients and clinicians, are partners in the construction of integrated practice. More simply put, a systemic clinician will invite the patient presenting with 'heartache' to look at the symptom from a variety of stances (broken heart, heavy heart, divided heart,

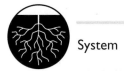 System

A system is any unit structured by and around feedback (Bateson 1972) and made up of interacting parts which mutually influence one another, forming patterns of behaviour and communication. When two or more people interact, they are involved in a joint construction of actions and meanings. This relationship is an evolving one, with each person influencing the other and being in turn influenced by the other's responses and actions. Any action is viewed as a response and any response can be conceptualised as an action.

cupid's dart). It is not only (trained) experts that are expected to sort out the broken hearts, but it is for the patient – the 'expert by experience' – and relevant others to join forces with clinicians. This process of jointly questioning the symptom is central to systemic practice. Of course many patients (and professionals) are closely wedded to the idea that only through a thorough analysis of cause will a solution be found. Often all that is revealed by this archaeological dig for causes is the cause of that cause . . . and so on. The question: 'What does your wife do when you get a bout of tummy pain?' may initially seem a less important question than finding the result of yet another endoscopy. Yet, it is surprising how often the patient – and the clinician – becomes more interested in the new question and possible answers:

> *She gets very worried by my stomach pains. She has all sorts of remedies that she tries on me . . . learnt them from her mother . . . . Mind you, it didn't help her mother – she died from a cancer of the pancreas that the doctors ignored for ages.*

Positivism and linear causality

Positivist science has delivered many outstanding achievements and continues to be a powerful tool in understanding our world. It is essentially based on the notion of linear causality, with events or outcomes being understood in terms of: A causes B, B causes C, and so on. If there is something not functioning as well as it should, then it is our natural tendency to find out the cause(s) and, if necessary, work back to the original cause. This approach has a firm hold on current health care practices, both in physical and psychological health camps. Indeed it is now well embedded in popular thinking: 'If only you had the time for me to tell you more about my childhood then I think you might understand why I am like this' or 'It's all because of the accident ten years ago'.

Valuable though this model is, it also has serious limitations, particularly in the increasingly multidimensional and multicontextual worlds we inhabit. Thinking that

Perspectives on pain

Take the next three patients presenting with some form of physical pain. Before being tempted to examine them physically, consider doing the following:

*   Ask who else, near or dear, knows about the pain, or perhaps even more interestingly, who near or dear does *not* know about the pain.
*   Ask what your patient believes that person thinks is the 'cause' of the pain, or why you think they don't know about it.
*   Ask your patient why that person holds that belief.

Then do whatever you normally do during a consultation.

one event leads, in a straight line, to another event often seems to run counter to our own experience where we find it impossible to disentangle the many different factors and their sequence in causing specific outcomes.

Some philosophers are still arguing as to what came first – the chicken or the egg. Think of the last argument you had with your partner, child or parent. Who started it and what was it about? Was it what they said or was it about what you had said previously, or was it really about something someone else had said to you just before the argument? And how did you learn to fly off the handle? Isn't that what your father used to do in similar situations? As you can see, once you start looking it can be tricky to see where the dance started and it is often not helpful to lay 'blame' at anyone's door. It is the mutual steps that often count for more. Of course this does not let anyone off the hook for violence or abuse but it does suggest that we need to be more cautious about statements like A caused B.

Systemic practitioners do not believe that it is always useful or indeed possible to establish the 'truth' about who or what caused a particular outcome, whether a physical symptom or a relationship issue. When mum and dad are involved in a major argument and ask their 3-year-old onlooking son who started it (the chicken or the egg?), this 'referee' will find it difficult to blow the whistle on either parent. This has, in part, to do with loyalty issues in what tends to be a classic 'no win' situation. It also has to do with the virtual impossibility of establishing 'scientifically' what came first. Clinicians are no more privileged to know 'the truth' than little 3-year-old Azeem. And when it comes to undertaking some therapeutic work with the parents, they often find themselves in precisely the same uncomfortable referee position. Instead of being fascinated by theories about causation, systemic practitioners are curious about outcome:

> *I notice you have plenty of arguments and they all end in tears. What would you have to do differently now for there to be no tears at the end? What could you say or do now? What could she do or say now?*

The limits of linear thinking

Much has been written on this subject. One of the clearest accounts comes from one of the smartest generalists writing today (McWhinney 1995), who offers a very useful overview on the development of our current scientific and cultural context. He is particularly good at pointing out the arbitrariness of many of the categories that we devise, quoting Wordsworth in his poem 'The Tables Turned':

> *Our meddling intellect*
> *Misshapes the beauteous forms of things:*
> *We murder to dissect.*

It seems that we humans love to try to divide up the world and categorise it. In this process we lose something of the beauty of the whole, and the more complex way in which the parts connect and influence each other.

Health care systems and mechanisms of change

Health – and therefore health care systems – is a critical political issue for most governments. The pace of change and political pressure on Western health care systems has grown steadily in the last decade or so. Tensions between central control and local autonomy, between free markets and state intervention, between the voices of local people, front-line workers, experts and politicians all seem ever more stark. A whole new language has sprung up, of 'total quality management', 'human resources', 'stakeholders', 'partnerships', 'performance management', 'outputs', 'clinical governance'. Many of these words speak to the old contexts of linear causality and individuality. The working model is very mechanical: if we attend to inputs (materials, finance, technologies) and improve the processes (performance management, learning programmes, quality standards and targets) then we will get 'better' outputs (waiting lists, hospital league tables, less complaints).

However, almost in response to this notion of the system as machine, there has been born another set of words and phrases: 'whole systems working', 'primary care collaboratives', 'learning organisations' and 'complexity management'. There is a genuine renewed interest in patients as 'partners in service design', or 'experts by experience', all equally worrying neologisms though hopefully new practices!

Systems theory has a great deal to say about the relation of one part of a system to another part and this makes good intuitive sense. In mental health care, for example, we seem to be strikingly good at designing separate bits of the system. We invent 'assertive outreach teams', 'early crisis intervention teams', other assessment and treatment teams, and primary care mental health teams. We seem to be much less good at designing integrated systems that make sense to users or connect in meaningful ways.

Systemic practitioners are not interested in coercing patients to meet the recommended standards, or hit the evidenced-based targets. They do not spend time outlining the performance management response if the patients fail to reach the standard. A systemic response would be to try to discover the beliefs and organising ideas of the patient; to explore the context that keeps them from changing; to invite them to look at the possibilities from other perspectives; and to reflect with them about the advantages and disadvantages of movement. A systemic practitioner might be just as interested in the relation of the patient to other individuals in their living context, searching for and finding ways of bringing them into the conversation.

Systemic practice emphasises the collaborative nature of the consultation between patient, family and clinician. The focus is not only on pathology and problems, but also on the patient's resources and strengths. Treatment and management plans are worked out in partnership – 'co-constructed' as it is termed. The clinician does not provide quick fixes but elicits the patient's ideas, working out joint solutions.

Before giving you a prescription for the latest antidepressant, I would like to find out a bit more about your own strengths in battling depression. If you look back over the past two weeks – have there been times when you have been less depressed? When has that been and what's your explanation? What did you do that made it more tolerable? Could you do more in the future of what you felt was helpful then again? What strengths are there in your family that have seen them and you through difficult times? How do others around you manage not to get depressed?

Complexity theory

There is a new movement afoot! Complexity science and theory have taken off from physics and mathematics and are beginning to find a new home in health care, amongst other places (Plsek and Greenhalgh 2001, Plsek and Wilson 2001, Zimmerman *et al.* 2001). Leaving on one side the argument about whether complexity science is a science in the positivist sense of the word, there is no doubt that complexity theory offers some great metaphors for thinking about change in health care systems. Put simply, complexity thinkers argue that most health care interactions and systems are complex. They do not follow the old linear rules. Very few interactions in health care are in the simple zone where there is a high level of certainty about an intervention and a high degree of agreement about which intervention to use. Most inter-actions have little certainty and exist in the complex zone. For example, change in health care systems is closer to throwing birds than throwing stones. You can make up some basic organising rules about how birds should fly, but where the bird lands is partly up to the bird. This is one of the reasons why general guidelines are so rarely of much help: they define and then abstract specific circumstances. Yet, patients bring all of their wonderful chaotic 'mess' with them: their beliefs, their families, their uncertainties and their muddles. Guidelines are tools designed for the high ground of technical rationality not the swamp where most primary care occurs (Schon 1983)! We have to relinquish the machine metaphor which suggests that if we control the inputs and the processes tightly enough, then we can ensure the quality of the outputs (clinician behaviour, diabetic control). Complexity enthusiasts point out that this doesn't seem to be working in health care and they have suggested a new way of thinking and behaving more effectively in complex systems (see also an interesting website www.complexityprimarycare.org).

Translated to the level of health systems change it might go something like this:

> *Before offering an intervention I thought up earlier, perhaps you could tell me about some of the things you are already doing which already point in the direction we have been outlining? Why do you think you have been able to do those but not this? What might need to happen for it to be possible to move in that direction?*

The changing nature of primary care

Over the past decades there have been many significant changes in primary care. Some themes emerge that have reasonable cross-cultural reliability. Primary care has moved centre stage in many health care systems. The units of delivery – the health centres – are getting larger and more complex. They are also undergoing management changes. Information technology is a key feature of modern practice with the computer the third participant in most consulting rooms. In paperless practices new issues of data protection and confidentiality are emerging.

Appreciative inquiry

The traditional approach to change management follows the medical model: to examine the problem, to make a diagnosis and to prescribe a treatment. Sensible though this may seem, it is also true that by paying attention to problems we risk amplifying them. Appreciative inquiry (Cooperrider 1990) proposes that we look for what works, for success rather than for failure. This approach has been developed to manage organisational change. Its principles are simple:

- Do more of what works (rather than doing less of something you do not do well)
- Appreciate, magnify and value the best of what is
- Get a vision of 'what might be'
- Get into conversations of 'what should be'.

In practice, each team member is asked to describe a time when he or she feels the team really performed well and what the circumstances were at the time. Members are asked to describe when and why they were proud to be a team member. They then are encouraged to state what (and why) they valued most about being a member of the team (Hammond 1996).

The primary care population is changing too. Chronic disease management and the challenges – and pleasures – of old age are an increasing feature in primary care and as a consequence so are specialisation and multidisciplinary and collaborative team working. There is also a shift towards population-based and proactive organisation of care. This is only a small sample of the changes that are occurring world wide in primary care. Needless to say, in this climate of seemingly continuous change it has often been difficult for clinicians to focus on their primary task: addressing their patients' bio-psycho-social needs (Bloch 1987).

The computer as a member of the consultation

The new flat computer plasma screens have turned out to be far more useful members of the consulting team than the immovable clunky old screens. A gentle push and the screen is turned towards the patient. Clinician and patient can jointly look at the display, whether previous consultation notes, letters or the family tree. In this way some aspects of the patient's story are externalised, 'out there', rather than remaining simply in the clinician's head, ready for joint exploration.

Systemic practice is enormously helpful in navigating the changing territory of primary care as a system, whether it is looking outward from the practice at new responsibilities to work with other agencies, or whether it is looking at the team in terms of collaboration with a mental health worker. It would seem that patients are at some level more in control of their own illness. Patients are experts, experts by experience, and they can support and teach other patients. This is happening in the fields of arthritis and mental health. DAPHNE is a programme for turning patients with diabetes into diabetologists themselves – so that it is the patients who make the decisions, with the professional becoming a source of support and advice, rather than remaining the only expert or leader.

Next please ...

Mrs A has a relapsing and moderately severe depressive illness. She also has osteoarthritis and heart disease. She also turns out to be an expert knitter of jumpers and knowledgeable on the subject of flowers. Responses to her difficulties included knitting jumpers for a member of the practice and putting her in touch with a lifelong learning coordinator who helped her find a place at a local college where she participated in a class on horticulture. The practice has an extensive network of contacts with other agencies. The local gym and the arts studio were particularly useful. The practice were comfortable with this matrix approach which generated solutions in a variety of ways.

Next please ...

Nancy was the counsellor for the primary care team counselling scheme. The practice and Nancy both wished to avoid replication of a 'shifted outpatient' model of practice and spent much time in the first five months working out a collaborative relationship that would be mutually beneficial. This involved sitting in on each other's practice, teasing out the different paradigms of the professionals, working on information systems, debating issues of confidentiality, practising a variety of ways of working from formal referrals to regular consults and corridor conversations.

Systemic thinking is enabling and encouraging in a time of change. The systemic practitioner has the freedom to step onto any place on the map of change, then see, hear and feel the differences, facilitating new perspectives and other frames, as well as engendering optimism. Sometimes nothing changes but the problem is seen in a new light.

Ingredients of the systemic approach

2

This chapter covers:
- ○ Systemic headaches
- ○ Bio-psycho-social approaches
- ○ The systemic zoom lens
- ○ Key systemic terms and definitions
- ○ Cultural considerations
- ○ Narrative ideas

Headaches: for patients and clinicians

Given the changing political health contexts outlined in the previous chapter, it is somewhat reassuring that patients, or 'service users' as current fashion requires us to call them, have changed relatively little. Their presentations have remained the same: they come with minor and major headaches; it sometimes feels that they come too late or too often; they come full of pain and they can sometimes become, if we are honest with ourselves and take note of our own feelings, a 'pain' to us. We sometimes still rate them as 'compliant' or 'difficult', as 'deserving' or 'demanding' – or plainly 'impossible'. Some make our heart sink and others make our heart bleed. They turn up, alone or with their families, with minor and major ailments. If they know that we find them or their ailments tiring, our patients learn the language to engage us again – and we have them, we have each other, for life.

General practice can seem 'like the therapeutic contract from hell', the perfect place for 'ultra brief, ultra long therapy' (Launer 1996). People can come any time, as often as they like, but there is never enough time to see them properly. Patients that present primarily with emotional problems can be a struggle. We may be tempted to label them as having 'mental health issues'. You may even find yourselves using words like 'functional' or even the curious term 'supra-tentorial', implying that these symptoms are imagined or somehow less real because you cannot identify the pathology, the damaged tissue. These patients often feel particularly demanding, and we may wish to refer them on, first to the practice counsellor or, better still, to some specialist psychologist or psychiatrist elsewhere. Some of us may even tell ourselves 'I don't do mental health problems'. However, between 30 and 60 per cent of all consultations in general practice are either directly about mental distress or contain significant psychological issues. And it has repeatedly been shown (Balint 1957, Elder and

Holmes 2002) that using a psychological perspective pays off when working in primary care. It provides new and useful insights, but it can also be very time consuming and there is a temptation to leave such work to the 'experts'. Nothing would seem more overwhelming to an already pressurised front-line clinician than having to listen endlessly to a patient's unpacking of their entrenched problems – and this within the confines of a '10 minutes per patient' time slot. It is hardly surprising that primary care workers generally avoid such activities. But it is not an impossible task to connect usefully with our patients' personal or relationship distress. All that is needed is a framework and appropriate techniques that can be adapted to primary care settings.

Where is the pain? And whose pain is it, anyway?

Next please . . .

Mr A first saw his GP, Dr B, because of back pain. After some investigations 'nothing much' had been discovered. Both doctor and patient put the symptoms down to stress at work. Mr A seemed 'compliant' and agreed to take some medication and to follow his doctor's advice to 'take it easy'. There seemed to be some initial improvements, but five weeks later the problems were back – in the back. Dr B tried a new course of tablets, but there was no change. Mr A said that the pain was now 'really getting me down'. Dr B thought that a course of antidepressants might be the answer, but when Mr A returned a week later, he said that the tablets were making him 'very dopey' and a bit sick. Dr B reassured his patient, but Mr A returned two weeks later with much the same complaints. A new antidepressant was promptly prescribed, but with no better outcome. Dr B then made an appointment for Mr A to see the practice counsellor. Mr A went once and then told Dr B that he did not want to have further 'sessions' as he did not think he was depressed or 'mental' – he just had terrible back pain.

Anyone working in primary care will have had their fair share of patients like Mr A – there are plenty of Mr and Ms As, just as there are many Dr Bs. These patients make

Compliance, adherence and concordance

It won't surprise readers to hear that, unlike Dr B, we generally prefer the term concordance to that of adherence or compliance. You may feel that moving the language from compliance to concordance is pure political correctness but there is a point – compliance is a word embedded in the idea that powerful doctors tell obedient patients what to do. 'Our job to make the plan, their job to follow it.' We know, however, that patients have minds of their own. How many prescriptions are never even taken to the pharmacy? Concordance has within it the idea that it is only by discovering where the patient is 'coming from', their beliefs and attitudes to whatever plan is being constructed, that you have a chance of successfully carrying through the plan. How often have you decided to be 'non-compliant' with a government diktat? Now, wouldn't you like a government that adopted an end-user-centred approach to change?

their clinicians feel bad and the clinicians make their patients feel no better. Let us imagine that Mr A had met Dr C, a GP with systemic glasses and contextual vision.

New lens please . . .

Mr A first saw his GP, Dr C, because of back pain. In the first consultation Dr C gave the patient a thorough physical examination. She said that she had felt some tense and painful back muscles and that she was going to prescribe some tablets to ease the pain. She predicted that this was only going to make a little difference and that one also needed to think about reducing 'some of the pressures' that were converging on the back. Dr C asked about physical pressures first and followed this up by asking Mr A about 'other pressures'. Mr A talked about work and both doctor and patient agreed that it was difficult to know how to reduce this pressure, given that Mr A had just landed this job, after a long period of unemployment. Dr C did not advise her patient to 'take it easy' at work, as this did not seem to be an option at this time. Instead she asked: 'Is there anyone who can take some of the pressure off your back?' Mr A seemed puzzled and Dr C explained: 'Well, I mean like family or friends?' Mr A then spoke about his wife and how she felt very burdened by having to look after her dementing mother. He said she was therefore 'very busy' and that this meant that he had to be much more involved with their teenage children: 'This is quite stressful'. When asked who he could talk to about how stressful things were for him, Mr A replied 'There isn't really anybody'. Ten minutes were up and Dr C asked Mr A to come back the following week.

It is hardly surprising to learn that the symptoms and problems of one person can affect other family members – and, that the responses of those near and dear significantly impact on the physical and psychological welfare of this person. Using a relationship lens opens up new perspectives that can be helpful.

Relationship lens please . . .

One week after Dr C first inquired about Mr A's back pain there had been some very modest improvement. Dr C said that continuing to take the tablets would make some difference, but that one would need to look at all the pressures to see whether some additional relief could be brought. She took a piece of paper and drew a big circle on it: 'Mr A, let's imagine that's you . . . now let's draw all the pressures that are operating on you'. Mr A mentioned his job, his ill father, his physical health, his back, his financial problems. 'And when you are really stressed, where do you feel it?' Mr A pointed to his back. 'So, what would relieve that pain . . . if you could take away one of the pressures, which one would it be? Or if you could share one of the pressures with someone else, how would you go about it? Show me on the piece of paper . . . .' Both Dr C and Mr A studied the piece of paper as if it was real. 'Maybe my wife could help me with my father?' Dr C: 'So, how would or could you talk about this to her?'

The person, the family and others

There are many stresses on Mr A and all may be important. But in some ways the relevance of family is unique. It is the major source of both social support and personal stress. It affects the individual's health, which in turn affects the family health. The family is also the source of the genetic and cultural material that makes up the individual. And the family is also a major ally of the health professional. The health of families in turn is influenced by the larger community, of which they are part. And families, in turn, affect the health of the community. Unhappy families are also often illness-prone families. The shortcomings of the traditional biomedical model become particularly evident when managing patients from socially disadvantaged families, or from different ethnic backgrounds which subscribe to very different illness concepts.

Next please ...

Mrs Y is an Iraqi woman with chronic shoulder pain. On physical examination it is evident that the muscles of her right shoulder are overdeveloped, probably as a result of chronic tension. She wants physiotherapy or massage to get rid of the tension. Further exploration reveals a history of personal torture in Iraq, witnessing the murder of her best friend and little daughter, daily nightmares and flashbacks. She also talks about domestic violence from her husband who himself was a victim of torture. Will physiotherapy of the right shoulder make things 'better'?

Next please ...

Ms P is 33 and has five children from three different partners. She has one child with severe asthma, which she controls very well. Her second son has moderate learning difficulties and is encopretic. She has had problems with alcohol in the past, resulting in her children being taken into care. When she doesn't drink she is an excellent mother; in fact she copes with more than you think you could. She is drinking again.

Bio-psycho-social approaches

Patients such as Mrs Y and Ms P leave the individual clinician feeling very ineffective and longing for new ways or 'magic' insights to proceed more helpfully in the consultation. The traditional medical model singularly fails to help in this more complex territory. One of the more successful ideas has been the bio-psycho-social approach which begins to make connections between illness, social environment and lifestyle (Engel 1977, 1980, Bloch and Doherty 1998). It looks at more than just the patient who has come to see the doctor: problems are not viewed as simply residing inside one person but as being connected with who and what is around that person. Symptoms and problems can be triggered or maintained by a spouse or another family member and thus be part of a family 'dis-ease'. Of course, they can often be triggered by social stresses outside the family.

Some thoughts on the word 'family'

The term 'family' is now open to many interpretations. Gone are the times when it implied a two-parent, heterosexual couple, ideally with two children and two pets, with the woman primarily the 'homemaker' and the man the 'breadwinner', drawing on occasional backup from grandparents who live within walking distance. Such a picture marginalises and excludes the nowadays more frequently encountered family forms, such as childless couples, single parents with children, reconstituted families, gay or lesbian couples and unattached persons. 'Family' in this book refers to many different forms of committed relationships and friendships. It describes any group of people who nurture each other emotionally or physically. Whatever the current 'family' may consist of, whether defined by genetic bonds or other emotional ties, whether lone parents, homosexual or heterosexual couples, blended or reconstituted families, large extended kinship networks or whatever, almost everyone relates to some kind of 'family'. Moreover, everyone has a family of origin, whether biological or not. This initial family contributes to the health of the individual, socially and emotionally and often genetically. If this is the case, then why not use the 'family', or the relationship context, as a resource in helping the individual patient who presents in primary care with a request for help?

Bio-psycho-social (BPS)

Bio-psycho-social is an important phrase that needs careful use, as it is easy to apply it glibly. It means the integration of biological ideas with thinking of the individual within the context of the family and community. A BPS clinician will deal with all the interlocking ideas in one consultation. A patient with ulcerative colitis will learn about the medical control of her symptoms in relation to how to function at her job and will learn to pay attention to how she manages anger and stress with her family and how that affects her diarrhoea. It is as though each of the dimensions is a circle which increasingly overlaps with the others. It is an especially important concept for thinking about relapsing conditions like asthma and irritable bowel syndrome. Like all ideas it has been found to have limitations. It pays little attention to political issues or issues to do with power, race, class or gender. But it is a pretty good place to start. One of the authors was lucky enough to sit in on tutorials with Engels in almost the last year of his teaching career. His mantras have always stuck: 'Never ask all your usual questions and then turn the spotlight on relationships or feelings. Always integrate questions from the three domains.' So obvious – and so easily forgotten!

Gender issues

In the systemic field, many early descriptions of family life and problems failed to take into account the fact that men's and women's experience of life is radically different. It was as though families were unisex creations. Feminist writers (Goldner 1988, Walters *et al.* 1988, Perelberg and Miller 1990, Hare-Mustin 1991, Burck and Daniel 1995) emphasise that clinicians need to take into account the different socialisation processes of men and women and how family life is shaped by culturally shared discourses of gender. They also draw attention to how language and speech patterns are gendered.

Gender differences also vary within different cultures and are subject to cultural expectations. In many societies male patriarchy is dominant and, when met by women's increased desire for equality, it can create particular dynamics in marriage and intermarriage. Perhaps it is only a myth that dominant-culture men are attracted to allegedly 'submissive' East Asian women, in search of a fading male sense of power in the age of feminism. The honeymoon phase, however, often does not last long.

Using a systemic zoom lens

'Thinking families' means studying and treating problems within the context(s) in which they occur. It is possible to do this with just one person actually present in the consulting room (Jenkins and Asen 1992, Boscolo and Bertrando 1996). Using the family lens is a way of getting patients to see their symptoms and themselves in a broader context: that of their immediate relationships, whether these involve a partner, family or significant others. Instead of narrowly focusing on a patient's head, for example, and the aches 'inside' it (intrapsychic), the clinician and the patient both step back and examine things 'outside' it. It is a bit like zooming back to a wide-angle position with a camera that was closely focused on one object. In this way the field of observation is gradually widened and enlarged. This is not to say that one always needs to place symptoms immediately in the wider context, thus ignoring the often crucially important individual details. It is of course very important to look closely at the presenting problem, otherwise one might miss vital clues. But there are obvious dangers with tunnel vision: you cannot see what is going on outside the tunnel. The 'zoom lens approach' is very different – it is 'environmental', it is dynamic and does not passively wait for the light at the end of the 'tunnel' to emerge.

This approach not only makes it possible to examine the symptom closely, but connects it with the context(s) within which it occurs, whether that is the family, other significant relationships, a particular neighbourhood or even a (sub)culture. It is an approach that allows flexibility by creating the possibility of new perspectives or 'frames' within which to view the patient and his symptoms, helping the clinician to remain flexible, curious and interested in the patient's predicament. Patients like learning about lenses.

Readers must be more than familiar with getting stuck within the first few minutes of a consultation, wondering why it does not seem to be making sense. The affect of the patient does not seem to 'fit' with the symptoms. In an inspired moment one can ask: 'How did you come to the decision to make an appointment today?', to which the response might be: 'Oh I didn't, my mother made it for me. She is always worrying about these things.' This response can lead the clinician to feel that light is dawning, with a mild relief that there is now some direction. 'So, what is it that your mother is most anxious about? And do you share that concern? How can we help your mother to stop worrying about this?'

Next please . . .

Mr N came with his wife to seek advice about his catastrophic thinking. Since having ME some years ago he had a tendency to get 'depressed' if the slightest thing went wrong and would very rapidly (within minutes) feel suicidal. His wife was terrified: 'It's as if he can't see the broader picture'. His tunnel vision was redefined as tunnel thinking. He recreated a wide-angle view by carrying around a laminated yellow card which said 'WHOA'. This, he said, helped put on the wide-angle lens and kept him safe.

It is surprising – but it should not really be – how a clinician's interest usually has a positive effect on the patient. In looking for connections between their symptoms and life situation, the patient is engaged in a process of questioning: questioning the symptoms, questioning themselves, and questioning those around them. This is a useful shift because all illnesses or problems tend to have some effect on the whole family. What at first sight seems to be one person's problem is frequently a family affair.

Patients' stories

One way of looking at primary care consultations is to think of patients telling their problem stories.

Next please . . .

Ms T consults her GP for recurring headaches. She has had these symptoms for the past six months. Recently she changed her doctor because she felt that he was unable to help her. She maintains that this doctor had 'tried his best', but that 'he didn't know what was wrong'. He had eventually sent her to various specialists, including neurologists, with second and third opinions confirming that there was 'nothing physically wrong'. Ms T said that none of these investigations had explained or cured her headaches. When her GP suggested that she should see a psychiatrist she decided to register with a different practice. Ms T feels that she has not been listened to or been understood.

Ms T tells her story about how her headaches were managed. It is not a success story. Her story, her narrative, is a highly subjective one and her doctor tells quite a different story when he discusses her 'case' with a colleague:

Zoom lens or wide-angle lens?

Here are two possible seeds you may wish to plant:

1 Pick two patients whom you know fairly well and who present with rather non-specific symptoms. Next time you see them:
   - Use a 'zoom lens' approach: focus tightly on the presenting problem, then zoom back (in your mind) and see the symptom in context, the person in context, the family in context. Zoom back far enough so that you can see yourself in the picture. Then zoom in again.
   - Find out, in detail, when the symptom occurs and what interactions take place around that time (see Chapter 4 for some useful phrases to use when questioning the symptom).
   - Speculate on how your patient's symptoms affect the family members or significant others – and how each family member (significant others) may affect the symptoms.
2 In the next surgery try to ask at least half the patients that you see how they came to make the decision to come today.
   - 'I was wondering how you decided to come today rather than a few days ago or in a few days' time?'
   - 'How did you arrive at the decision to see me today?'
   - 'Was anyone else involved in making the decision to come today?'
   - 'Who made the decision to come today (when there are two people seeing you)?'

Ms T is a woman who somatises her own unhappiness. There are no organic causes for her recurrent headaches. I have investigated her symptoms extensively, she has seen a number of specialists, there is nothing physically wrong with her. Despite my continuous reassurances she insists that her headaches are still there. I believe they are a symptom of her underlying emotional problems and this is why I referred her to a psychiatrist.

You, the reader, could probably tell a different story about these two stories. The reason why you can do so is that you are in what is called a 'meta-position' in relation to the story told: you are outside the interaction(s) between doctor and patient. Maybe you would want to retell the story with a hero, the doctor, and a villain, the patient. Or perhaps the other way round. Or perhaps you just see them as hopelessly feeding into one another. Storytelling is as old as mankind. It is the way we have always made sense of our experiences and how we create our world(s). It is the way we communicate and how we affect one another.

Stories are now more fashionably called 'narratives' and there is a whole new field of narrative-based practices emerging in different medical and therapeutic settings, including in primary care (Greenhalgh and Hurwitz 1998, Launer 2002). Patients tell their own experiences in narratives or have their experience told as stories by others. These 'dominant narratives' (White and Epston 1990) may not fit with what patients themselves have actually experienced. In fact, they may even contradict their experiences. The systemic narrative approach attempts to enable patients and families to generate and evolve new stories and ways of interpreting events to make sense of their experiences. Patient and clinician 'co-evolve' or 'co-construct' a new 'story' so that a new focus emerges.

Next lens please . . .

Ms T's new GP asks her about patterns of family health and responses to illness. To do this he draws together with Ms T, on a piece of paper, a family tree. Ms T remembers that her mother developed what she called 'tension headaches' shortly after Ms T's birth, some 21 years ago. The GP asks Ms T whether she thought that there was a connection between her and mother's headaches and Ms T suddenly remembers that her headaches started one month after she had a termination of her pregnancy. At this point the GP refrains from interpreting the possible link between this event and the onset of the headache and makes another appointment for his patient: 'Perhaps you want to come back some time next week – maybe you might even bring your mother, but I leave it to you. You decide whether this might be useful.' The patient accepts the appointment. The headache is no longer just in her head, it has become connected with events and people around her. A new story emerges. Next time she brings her mother and they begin to discuss who and what gives each of them headaches. Ms T's headache has become the family headache.

A patient's headache not infrequently becomes a 'headache' to doctors and other clinicians, particularly when no immediate physical or obvious psychological causes can be found. What clinicians do to investigate headaches varies a great deal. If a doctor comes fresh from hospital medicine, he may, influenced by his recent clinical experience of severe cases, give undue weight to the possibility of this being a brain lesion. Another doctor with, say, a keen interest in psychological medicine

Storytellers

We are all storytellers. And we often use stories to tell others about ourselves and our families, and to give others ideas about who we are. If you cast your mind inwards you may identify a number of family stories that have become 'standards' in your repertoire. Some may be from your family of origin, others from a family you are busy constructing now. These stories help us to define and sometimes confine us. Therapy is partly about identifying these stories and seeing whether new ones are possible.

Elizabeth Stone (1989), an historian by training, wrote a classic account of the way we use and abuse these stories in the endless construction and reconstruction of the self. It is well worth getting hold of if you can.

would be more likely to attribute emotional causes to the headache. A health visitor, in turn, with direct experience of family dynamics, may suggest a diagnosis of 'family stress'. Taking a good history of the presenting symptom or problem is important, no matter what your persuasion or bias. How detailed such an examination is in the first consultation will depend on a variety of factors, but above all it will depend on the clinician's hunches. Experience, knowledge of that particular patient and some of their life circumstances, intuition, a whole range of 'soft' data and informed guesses go to make up hunches. Acting on your hunches is good practice when you look for confirmation or refutation of your ideas and hypotheses, rather than simply mistaking the hunches for the truth.

A way into all this through the symptoms

The majority of patients present with what they regard as physical symptoms, and the clinician will therefore have to weigh up to what extent these need to be investigated. Few patients object to having their blood pressure taken, their fundi looked at and perhaps their eyesight tested. Being physically examined signals to many patients that they are being taken seriously, but it is also a good time to probe further if the clinician follows his hunch that there might be a 'family dimension' to the problem. Such probes mostly take the form of questions, some of which may be puzzling to the reader at this stage – they will be explained in Chapter 4. Take another patient who presents with headaches:

Learning to discover multiple perspectives

Choose one patient and their illness/problem 'story'. Invent a few alternative stories, perhaps the one the partner, the child or the grandfather might tell. Next time you see the patient ask what their partner/child/grandfather might have to say about the illness. Listen to your patient's narrative and compare – in your mind only – with your own stories.

- 'Who in your family knows about your headaches?'
- 'How are your headaches affecting members of your family?'
- 'What sort of responses do you get? Who is most sympathetic? Who least?'
- 'Who or what tends to make the headaches better?'
- 'Is there anything you can do to make them get better?'

And to a child:

- 'I wish your tummyache could talk to me. What might it say?'

These and other questions are aimed at introducing the context in which the headaches occur through the back door, as it were. The clinician is not suggesting that the patient's headaches are not real or implying that they are psychological, but is asking the patient to look at them in context, how they affect others and how others affect the headaches. The clinician also encourages the patient to examine their own coping strategies, sometimes asking: 'Do you have any theories yourself why you are having these headaches?' Often this question gets a patient to reflect aloud, which may lead to some useful exchange. At times the patient's sharp reply is as follows: 'No, I don't, you are the doctor! If I knew I wouldn't have come here in the first place. You are the expert, aren't you?'

This answer has, over time, silenced many a doctor. There is a reply, however:

'Yes, of course I am, but often patients have their own ideas and these are very important . . .'

Interventive, non-blaming approaches

Adopting a family approach does not mean that you should blame the family for being the cause of illness. It highlights that the family is often the 'site' at which the suffering takes place. The family systems approach is not really interested in finding a 'villain' or apparent cause for the dysfunction of an individual. Instead, it aims to promote change. It accepts that in many cases there is multiple causality and that, when it comes to human interactions, it is helpful to invoke the concept of 'circular causality'. When it comes down to it, it is quite impossible to determine whether Mrs X is so depressed because Mr X constantly nags her. Or whether he always has a go at her because she is depressing him so much.

The bio-medical model traditionally locates pathology *inside* a person. The family systems model is interactional and views problems as arising *between* people. The approaches are not mutually exclusive; on the contrary, they complement one another. All of us are the product of genetic and constitutional factors, past experiences, physical and social factors, and so on. And yet there can be little doubt that our current behaviours and problems are also related to forces operating in the present. Primary care workers need to address all aspects – past, present and future. This means being interested in asking three questions simultaneously: 'What went on *then*?' 'What's going on *now*?' 'What's possible in the *immediate future*?'

Many primary care workers tend to use a medical lens first. After all, that is what doctors and nurses have been trained to do. But if an interview keeps a tight medical focus at all times, the patient may feel like an object of investigation. This type of interaction may well be what patients have come to expect and at some level it may appear to be less threatening – to everyone concerned! Patients generally do not want to be passive subjects and systemic practitioners tend to believe that exploration through questioning leads to a reflective process, both in the patient as well as in the clinician. The process of finding out is often more important than being told some 'home truths', if indeed there ever is such a thing. The journey of getting to a destination is so often more exciting than being parked in a secure environment. Questions have the purpose of widening the field of observation and explaining the contextual function of symptoms: '*Why* now?' '*Who* suffers most or least as the result of the illness?' '*What* would happen if the patient got suddenly better?' '*What* are the positive effects of the symptom(s) on everyone?'

When it comes to the area of interpersonal relationships, a questioning approach is often very useful, helping patients to come up with their own explanations, even if this takes a bit of time. In this way the clinician becomes a catalyst, enabling patients to change their views and positions, at their own pace and in their own time.

The function of symptoms

Symptoms not only have causes, they also can be said to have 'functions'. This means that they can be useful and not just a nuisance. If there is marital conflict, a headache may be a welcome visitor, giving some kind of permission not to get involved in arguments: 'I'm sorry, I can't talk about this now, I've got a headache'. At the outset, the spouse may respond and accommodate as their partner is so 'unwell'. The headache could be said to have the function of creating some distance at awkward times – it can even stabilise a rocky marriage. However, after some time the partner often becomes increasingly irritated by the frequent headaches and a new set of problems may arise – which could be experienced as a game by the partner. But the headaches are real to the patient and not part of a conscious strategy to put some distance between them. This is often when real arguments start – and members of the primary care team may be drawn into this battle.

The patient's headaches then can also have a function in the context of the consulting room: they are the symptomatic person's ticket to having a sympathetic ear, more sympathetic than their partner's ear. This produces a dilemma: if you cure the headaches too quickly, then your patient's reason for seeing you will go. Your patient may need to find new ways to keep you engaged as a sympathetic helper, for instance by experiencing new symptoms or a sudden unexplained relapse. Whilst sympathetic ears can be seemingly good 'solutions' to allow patients to air their distress, they can also become problems in their own right when patients get addicted to the clinician's pair of ears.

Focusing on the symptom

Let us suppose the clinician cannot find anything physically wrong with a patient. Being aware that the patient wants something and feeling a need to give 'it', the clinician could prescribe some placebo. But it may be possible to give the patient a task instead:

I cannot find a physical reason at the moment, but that does not mean that there is no physical reason. Headaches are very tricky customers, they can be caused by all sorts of things, including stress and worry. I suggest you keep a diary about your headaches, day by day, when they occur, how long they last for, and what makes them better or worse. When you come back in a week's time we can both look at it together.

This is not just a simple time-buying device: the 'prescription' of focusing on the symptom is often very effective. First, it can provide useful information for the primary care worker who can see whether a hunch has been right or not. But, more importantly, the patient is turned into the investigator of their own aches and pains and thus becomes a collaborator in the diagnostic and treatment process. Armed with new information the patient may return in a week's time and they can both make sense of the data together. In this way the patient is not just the passive recipient of some diagnostic process or treatment, but becomes an active participant in it. The process of self-observation and the recording of onset, duration and circumstances of the symptoms often helps patients to make some important connections. If your patient returns and tells you that the headaches always happen at 8.30 p.m.,

Using diaries

Diaries are sometimes really useful in general practice. They feel a bit like a prescription with all that prescriptions imply about giving, making a plan, something that might help, a piece of paper, etc. They are a way of getting more information and, like every task, they are also a potential therapeutic intervention because they ask patients to reflect and observe what is happening. A diary can be used in at least the following three ways: (1) It allows you to ask questions indirectly. For example, 'I'd like to know more about Bill's headaches. Perhaps you and your husband could keep a diary of exactly when and how they start?'

(2) It allows the exploration of coping strategies: 'Could you keep a careful note of what you do to try and help him, and what sort of effect that has? This helps me to get your combined view of what is happening.' (3) It involves all the participants. Perhaps it feels like one of the parents or protagonists in the situation is not very involved. Asking them to be part of the task of completing the diary can be a way of involving them in the solution – if you change their steps chances are someone else's steps may change as well.

Here are two ideas to try:

- Ask two patients to keep a diary for the following week, recording precisely when symptoms occur, noting who is present and noting the effects on significant others. Discuss the observations during the next consultations. Allow the patient to draw all the conclusions.
- Keep a diary yourself of when *you* have remembered to use a systemic idea in a consultation and then speculate on why you did it then and not at other times. What helped you do it and what hindered you? What might make you more likely to use it again?

at about the time when her partner goes to the pub, then there is little that you need to explain! However, if you also discover that the patient consumes large quantities of chocolate around that time, then you need to revise your assumptions and look at cause and effect issues from a variety of different perspectives.

The family as a system

It is important to state that if we talk about the family as a 'system', this is merely a useful metaphor rather than some kind of real 'truth'. It is useful to look at the family as if it were a system, with different interacting parts, working according to some unwritten rules. Yet, we have to remember that it is the observer who constructs this picture and this also limits its usefulness. A particular characteristic of a system is the notion of boundaries. Again, this is merely a useful metaphor rather than a 'real' thing – useful in that it permits comprehension of family dynamics and can inform therapeutic *interventions*.

Two types of so-called 'boundary disturbances' are particularly important in the systemic therapies: boundaries that are deemed to be 'too weak' and those that are 'overly strong'. For example, a family with a seemingly impermeable boundary is likely to adapt poorly to the arrival of new members such as babies or boyfriends, and will be less tolerant of members such as adolescents moving out. Families with seemingly 'too weak' boundaries live in each other's pockets, being expert at mind-reading

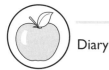

Diary

Prescribing a diary task is no different in many ways to prescribing a medicine. If you want the patient to do it then you are interested in achieving concordance. What ways are there to increase the likelihood of a patient using a diary and gaining useful insights?

Check interest in the idea before going further. If they are not ready for change then they are unlikely to do the diary – it won't be some people's preferred way.

- 'Being realistic, and on a scale of 1 to 10, how likely is it that you will be able to fill in a diary?'
- 'Do you think you are likely to fill a diary in?'
- 'What do you think of this as an idea?'

Have a copy of a diary with some examples of the sort of way you would like it filled in.

Check on literacy levels, as some 30 per cent of your patients may have trouble with reading or writing:

- 'Are you the sort of person that finds it easy writing things down or reading them? Or do you find difficulty with reading or writing?'
- 'Some people are great at writing things down, some people are better at talking! Which sort of person are you?'

and talking for one another. These so-called 'enmeshed' families have little differentiation between parents and children, few hierarchical structures and little private space for the individual family members. For example, when the parents always defer important decisions and ask their 4- and 6-year-old children for advice, then it could be said that the boundary around the parental subgroup is non-existent. The children are elevated into an executive position which is likely to result in more or less unstructured, if not chaotic interactions, with nobody 'in charge'.

This can present problems, though some family – and indeed some cultures – seem to be more tolerant than others of seeming 'chaos'. Most families, however, fall somewhere in the middle, with both enmeshed and disengaged patterns of communication present at specific times or in certain situations. Cultural patterns as to what the 'right' place for the child is vary enormously. In some cultures the first-born, particularly if a boy, may have a highly significant status. Of course, descriptions that use notions such as 'too weak' or 'too strong' are clearly based on normative assumptions and prejudices. Whilst common sense is based on such prejudices, with all its obvious advantages and disadvantages, political correctness obliges us to be reverent and pretend that we are open-minded, even-handed, neutral and neutred!

Next please . . .

Mrs L, in her late forties and very 'classy', talked to the practice nurse about her 14-year-old daughter Lisa. She was worried that Lisa had the beginnings of an eating disorder and she wanted some dietary advice. The practice nurse weighed Lisa and found that she was on the 25th percentile. Mrs L said that she and Lisa 'have no secrets from each other'. She described the family as being very 'open', everyone telling everyone else their concerns and worries. 'We always keep all the doors open . . . our bedroom door, the doors of the children's rooms . . . even the bathroom door doesn't close properly. We don't believe in locks.' The practice nurse asked: 'So, what happens if you want to be private?' Mrs L seemed alarmed: 'Why would anybody do anything in private? We all trust and respect each other.'

In this family, privacy was viewed as a crime, a betrayal of the family. Is Lisa's emerging eating disorder her protest against an unboundaried family? Families are highly complex systems with many subgroupings, within the nuclear and extended context. Most families are not static entities but function differently at different times, with some flexibility all round. For example, on occasions the parental couple may operate as 'husband and wife' and at other times as 'parents'. Sometimes the children form a subgroup, ganging up against their parents. Occasionally cross-generational subgroups, such as mother–grandmother or child–grandfather, form temporary or permanent alliances with good or bad effects on the family dynamics.

Families, like other biological systems, are usually in a fragile homeostatic state which can be upset by illness, by addition or loss of a family member or many other stresses. In the face of a crisis the family may have to change to accommodate to the new situation: some roles may need to be allocated anew, the way family life is organised may have to change drastically. The homeostatic tendencies of families may work against making such changes and sometimes the solutions families try do not work to restore the balance as intended. It is frequently at this point that one or more family members decompensate and present at their doctor or primary care worker.

Boundaries

Boundaries are conceptual demarcations between or within systems and subsystems. They are determined by the invisible rules defining participation by family members in different types of interactions. Internal family boundaries are recognisable by the different rules governing behaviours within different family subsystems. The rules that apply to parental behaviours (parental subsystem) are usually different from those that apply to child behaviours (child subsystem). The boundaries between the family and the external environment are determined by family scripts, cultural practices and other contextual issues.

Family problems do not result from the behaviour of just one person, but they are connected with the way family members relate to one another. What each person does affects others and a chain reaction occurs which tends to follow a rather predictable path and to be extremely repetitive. Observing the part each family member plays in the chain of (family) events, under what circumstances they are set off and how they are maintained, provides useful information that can be helpful in putting a stop to the inevitable snowballing of problems.

Family styles

Families differ a great deal in the way they are organised: there are idiosyncratic and cultural differences and it is important for clinicians to be respectful of the way families live according to these (mostly unwritten) rules.

Next please ...

Mr H had been brought up by a succession of nannies. He hypothesised that a few minutes after being born, his mother had handed over 'that smelly and screaming baby' to the nanny. In subsequent years the only real contact he remembered with his mother was being 'presented to

Homeostasis

Homeostasis, or system stability, may be desirable or undesirable depending on context. For example, when a family system is facing a new phase in its life cycle which will lead to changes for family members, self-regulatory feedback can push the system towards a 'no change' reaction, in an attempt to preserve an earlier stability. On the other hand, a certain degree of internal stability is an essential condition for the optimal functioning of the family, allowing for beneficial growth.

*mum' after being bathed and perfumed. His mother had only encountered the child in a sani-
tised way – the perfect and aseptic baby and child. Preparatory and boarding schools had succeeded in keeping him at arm's length from his family of origin and the predictably chosen
exclusive university college had further contributed to the sense of splendid isolation. When he
presented to the primary care team with morbid fears about contamination, venereal disease
and other infections, his GP, Nigerian and from a closely knit family, had to bite his tongue to
stop being critical of a different (rather than odd) family.*

Next please ...

*One of the authors spent several months working as a paediatric junior doctor in New Zealand.
There was a measles epidemic in the mainly Maori population of the poorer part of the town. The
ward was filled with unwell rash-covered kids. On several occasions the staff, who were mainly
Pakeha (white), got in real muddles as children with the same surname, who were brothers or sisters, seemed to have two mothers. First-born children in many Maori families are brought up by
their grandmothers. This added a richness and complexity to the care of these children.*

The idea of family styles and types has had great utility over the years. Some
workers, however, have come to stereotype certain families, and the class and
cultural backgrounds they come from. As a result clinicians can be at risk of
disallowing certain ways of behaving or talking. Statements such as: 'This is the
way enmeshed families behave' need to generate doubt and caution in both listener
and speaker. It is2 important to recognise that no one set of people in a family is
the same as any other. Understanding this variation and retaining curiosity about
diversity remains a critical stance for any clinician.

Cultural considerations

Culture can be defined as a system of shared meaning, It is a complex construct
of socially transmitted attitudes, beliefs and feelings that shape behaviours, organise
perceptions and label experiences. Culture affects communication styles, gender and
family roles, and personal and group identity. It also affects the identification and
diagnosis of problems in the mental health arena, as well as the expectations of
service users and health professionals. People from different cultures express their
distress differently, with a great variation of what 'qualifies' as a mental health
issue or illness. In this sense culture constructs our identities and behaviours, whilst
at the same time we construct culture. In multicultural societies, cultures exist within
cultures and usually in hierarchical power relationships, with minority cultural
groups finding themselves marginalised and/or discriminated against.

Therapists need to be aware of these dynamics and how they impact on clients'
perceptions and use of therapeutic help offered. A culture-sensitive approach
demands the therapist's curiosity about, if not familiarity with, the cultural practices
of any given family. Furthermore, it requires both an ability to keep in mind the
multiple contexts of which the family is part, as well as a capacity to hold multiple
views of the 'problem' and the 'solutions'. Whilst culture contributes to pattern
people's lives, meanings and beliefs are subject to reworking within the host cultural
framework, with the therapist aiming to help the family and its individual members
to improve the ecological fit between the diverse cultural contexts.

Cultural considerations

When two people meet, they bring their respective cultures along with them, as surely as they bring their shadow. Only Peter Pan was able to lose his! Most primary care clinicians have been to university, unlike 60 per cent of the people they will see in their practices, and most earn considerably more than most of their patients. When those meeting also come from different ethnic groups and countries then the shadow cultures they bring can sometimes obscure the people themselves.

The Spirit Catches You and You Fall Down (Fadiman 1997) is an account of the collision of two cultures – the 'clash between a small country hospital in California and a refugee family from Laos over the care of Lia Lee, a Hmong child', diagnosed by the paediatricians as having severe epilepsy. Both protagonists, well meaning and genuine, arrive at a disasterous impasse based on lack of shared understandings. This book is but a glimpse of the rich field of trans- and cross-cultural health studies. This field endlessly underlines the need to retain uncertainty in trying to understand where the patient 'comes from' and 'what it all means to them'.

Cultural patterns show remarkable diversity. Take, for example, certain ideas about child-rearing. Some 100 years ago, in Great Britain, it was not uncommon for some young children to be 'adopted' by members of the extended family – childless uncles or aunts, for example. It was also much more common for the grandparents to live 'on site' and to contribute significantly to bringing up baby – or to interfere much more in their offspring's marital relationships. With the demise of the extended family in allegedly 'modern' Western societies, some of these intrafamily patterns are a thing of the past. Yet, in other societies and cultures the extended family is very much alive and has a major role in making – and breaking – family relationships. In many Afro-Caribbean families it is still not uncommon for grandmothers to be the main carers of young children. This is the norm and not some form of parental neglect. The role of fathers is also more marginal. Using standard cultural assumptions gets us nowhere when managing these families and their individuals.

The family dance

The family systems approach accepts that families have very different ways in which they live together. It adopts a non-judgemental stance: by understanding how each person's behaviour is choreographed by the whole family group, one can avoid siding with one member. Seeing one person's problems in context is like trying to work out the various steps in the 'family dance' (see also Chapter 10). If one person changes the steps, the rest need to change in some ways too: the dance can be altered by change in any one member. How the dance evolves is based on the intricate feedback loops that develop.

This idea of the 'dance' has proved one of the most useful of all the systemic ideas. It is often very easy to see some of the steps that we all take. Remember the film *Who's Afraid of Virginia Woolf?*, where the two protagonists slug it out in a bitter and passionate dance? How many times do you remember them going round the same loop of passion followed by the trivial trigger to violent argument, supplemented by drink? How many times have you watched while one of the practice team tries to introduce an innovative idea only to have it undermined by a team member who resists by restating their original position? Or was that the dance where a reasonable and necessarily cautious team member tries to get a young hothead to listen to the problems with a new idea rather than just see the potential?

It is generally accepted that it takes 'two to tango' and in most families the dance routines usually involve more than that. Some family jigs can involve the helpers as well, whether paediatricians, GPs, nurses, social workers or health visitors. What is fairly obvious is that one person alone cannot carry on an interaction all by themselves! There is always someone who encourages or reinforces certain behaviours and some kind of collaboration is necessary among family members to keep conflicts going, even if this is not conscious or deliberate. Yet, people often see themselves as merely reacting to others, rather than participating in the dances they are involved in. We have already talked about the limitations of the traditional linear model of causality and that systemic practitioners embrace a very different concept, that of circular causality. However, this also has its limitations, particularly since it cannot really account for power differentials that are so evident in society. These can be based on prejudices and oppressive practices in relation to stubbornly concrete social realities such as poverty, war or institutionalised discrimination on the basis of a person's gender, disability, sexual orientation, race or religion. These 'independent' realities are very real for many families, but they do not fit easily into the systemic circular frame.

The individual clinician's belief system, interviewing style and personality are important ingredients of any consultation – whatever the model used. The questions asked and the way in which a clinician probes will, to some extent, organise the patient's responses. The patient, in turn, 'feeds back' to the clinician, who will then respond to the patient's responses. In this way clinician and patient become an interacting 'system'.

Feedback

This term implies that an action or piece of behaviour by one person (A) has an impact on others (B) which may cause them (B) to respond in such a way that their behaviour may have a further impact on the behaviour of (A). This can be described as a loop of interaction. Feedback can be either positive, leading to change and variation, or self-regulatory (negative), producing stability and homeostasis. It is argued that systems function best when there is a balance between these two types of feedback. Self-regulatory feedback, which replaces the term negative feedback, leads to homeostasis and the restoration of the family's state of internal balance because the feedback loops tend to dampen any variation in initial input.

Spotting the dance

Tomorrow try and spot three 'dances':

1   One in your home life
2   One in the practice life
3   One in a patient's life.

The practice system

This idea of a 'dance' between patient and clinician is familiar to many primary care practitioners. What might be less familiar is the notion that not only the clinician but also the practice team and even the practice culture also contribute steps in the dance with the patient and their system.

Next please . . .

Mrs M, receptionist at the Couch End Group Practice, had, over time, developed a keen interest in the J family. They certainly were frequent attenders! It was always father who telephoned the surgery, usually at 9 a.m., requesting an urgent appointment for one of the children. A bit later the whole family would arrive – without father. Mother, grandmother and three young children would file in, one after the other. Mrs M was only too aware that the doctors and practice nurses were less than pleased to see this little procession yet again. On this occasion it was the middle child who was presented as the patient: 'He's been sick this morning!' Mrs M remembered that only a few days ago it had been the oldest who had been sick and a few days earlier it had been the youngest's turn. Both had made remarkably quick recoveries. In fact, the practice nurse had given strict instructions not to give this family another urgent appointment – and so had two of the doctors. Yet, here they were again, the 'family from hell' as they were fondly known in the group practice. Mrs M was fascinated that everyone in the household had come for each of the appointments – apart from father. She could not help but speculate about what might be going on in this family. Was he over-anxious? Was the mother not able to deal with minor physical problems? Why did they all come, including the maternal grandmother? What were the relationships between all these children and adults – and what were their relationships with the ever-absent father? Mrs M's brain was quite preoccupied with the different possible stories, but then had to stop as she had to take another urgent telephone call. We will therefore never know which of these stories she thought was the most likely – all we know is that she never shared her ideas with the practice nurses and doctors. What a shame!

Practice systems and family systems

Practice receptionists could be marvellous storytellers – if only clinicians were prepared to listen. However, they often think that it is neither their place, nor their role, to contribute to the understanding and management of families – even though they are often best placed to do so. It is worth noting that their perspectives are different and they can enlarge the frame (Cole-Kelly 1992).

By stepping back a bit further, another picture, another 'story', emerges: that of the interaction between father, family and the primary care team. Were Mrs M and the other receptionists really that neutral, or did they contribute to the plot, by providing appointments, giving in to the requests? And what was the role of the doctors? What did each person do to reinforce or sustain this 'problem-determined system' (Anderson *et al.* 1986)?

Systemic practitioners are interested in how relationship patterns evolve, not only inside a particular family, but also between the family and the primary care team (including the receptionist), and, last but not least, inside the team. This interest is not just academic, it also has pragmatic value. Generally we tend to think that if we can understand what goes on, then we can 'diagnose' what is 'wrong' and put it 'right'. Or that is at least how most of us have been trained to think. Yet, the reality is much more complex. The bad news is that we are not merely objective observers of the processes that go on within some systems. We speculate, we use our clinical prejudices, we construct some convenient hypotheses that – fingers crossed – we hope will 'fit'. But all too often we may just end up fitting our families and their individual members into our neat 'systems' and comfortable diagnoses. Just like Mrs M, we are part of the systems we 'observe'. It may be reassuring to her to view the scene from the safe distance of her reception desk. Yet she – along with so many secretarial and administrative staff in primary care teams – is playing a vital role. She responds to the feedback she receives from the clinicians and this generates a new feedback loop involving the family, who respond to her feedback; this, in turn, leads the clinicians to near-despair, taking out their irritation on the receptionist.

The receptionist as systemic practitioner?

Just imagine that the receptionist responds to a request for an appointment by saying, 'Supposing I did not have an appointment today to give you – what could you do instead?' 'OK, I understand that you could be annoyed, but what else could you do? Who or what could help you if the practice can't?'

We know, it sounds completely outrageous, but it makes you think. Receptionists are just as much a part of the system as clinicians and probably at least as skilful in working with people (on the way in) and patients (on the way out). So what training needs and what dialogues go with this realisation?

Read a paper

Dowrick (1992) has done a great job at untangling the relationship between a practice and a family such as the one described here. It is one of our favourite papers and a great introduction to the value of systemic ideas in primary care.

Spot a practice system

Pick a patient and their family who is frequently seen in your practice. In your head just start to wonder if the practice has developed any particular steps in relation to this family. How have you become part of the system?

If the idea intrigues you, you may wish to pull all the notes, start to 'do a Dowrick' on them. See if patterns of consulting changed at any stage, talk to one of the receptionists about their theories of why it is as it is. Be curious!

If you get really curious about the way family patterns develop then you might like to read another great book. Huygen (1978), a pioneering and strikingly meticulous Dutch GP, has written a small masterpiece. He has collected the medical histories of some 100 families with which he has been involved as a practitioner. He charted their consultation patterns, major life events, illnesses, births and deaths. Out of this mass of data Huygen has drawn some of the intricate patterns that emerge between families and specific illnesses, patterns of consultation and specific life events.

The evolution of systemic work

3

> This chapter covers:
> ○ The history of the systemic approach
> ○ A quick romp through some of the major schools of family and systemic therapy
> ○ The application of some of these ideas to primary care

Those familiar with the systemic field may well feel that there are other ways of telling its tale, but – as with all history – there are many different stories to tell about what may seem the same events. Skip this chapter if you think you know it all, but for those less familiar with the evolution of systemic theory and practice, it points at some 'milestones' along the journey, as well as clues to what has been considered important over the years. The history of family therapy theory and practice offers a rich tapestry of thoughts, discovery and an involvement with the cultural issues of recent decades in a way other psychotherapies do not. Like a living creature the theory and practice evolve together, and in a Darwinian way those ideas that work survive, evolve further and feel comfortable. If you are not familiar with the history, you could miss the colour and depth (Hoffman 2002).

It is now more than half a century since the anthropologist Gregory Bateson formed a team to study the communication patterns in families containing a schizophrenic member (Bateson *et al.* 1956). The group believed that in these families the ill person's thought processes were in part shaped through the bizarre communication requirements imposed by other members. Bateson's team also found that if the schizophrenic family member, hence called the 'identified patient' (i.p.), improved, the family would often decompensate. They speculated that the family 'needed' the i.p. to remain unwell, so that some kind of homeostatic state could be maintained. The team also observed that, when faced with therapeutic interventions, the family often resisted change. Over time Bateson and other workers developed the idea that the i.p. was really the family scapegoat, the victim of family dynamics and a collusive professional system. Logically, therapy aimed to 'liberate' the i.p. from this role and it resulted in practices that challenged the notion of the 'sanity' of the family (Cooper 1971).

The anti-psychiatry movement of the 1960s believed that it was the confusing communication patterns inside the family that caused the ill person's distorted perceptions (Laing and Esterson 1964). So, here was born the 'schizophrenogenic' mother, alongside the 'toxic family', with the parents themselves now scapegoated

Scapegoat practices

Scapegoating, or the blaming approach, has survived remarkably well into the new millennium. It is practised not only by some families and clinicians, but also by many health politicians! But when it comes to working with our patients, is it useful to view the mentally ill person just as the 'victim' of the family or society? It is certainly not a helpful stance when engaging carers and other family members in any therapeutic ventures. Yet most clinicians cannot help being influenced by the prevailing culture of blame. Furthermore, when focusing on power inequalities, poverty, stigma, social and racial discrimination it is difficult not to support the 'victim'. But are these practices empowering, or a further confirmation of a seeming 'failure' to be successful? There is more on this in Chapter 10.

for what had gone wrong with the i.p. Not surprisingly, there was little enthusiasm, in particular by parents, for this novel treatment called 'family therapy': they felt just misunderstood and blamed for their offspring's ill-health. As far as most parents were concerned, it was not the family which required therapy, but the patient. With hindsight, it would seem that these early excesses, inspiring though they seemed at the time, did little to establish the credibility and acceptability of systemic therapy.

Psychoanalytic family therapy

There were a number of parallel developments going on in the 1950s and 1960s. Most of the early pioneers in the field had been trained psychodynamically and those who were interested in seeing families developed *psychoanalytic family therapy* (Ackerman 1966). The approach focuses on painful emotions and unconscious processes, with the therapists bearing and managing those strong feelings that cannot be tolerated by the family, such as hostility, despair, futility and fear. The theory was that this 'containing stance' would allow family members to retrieve and reintegrate split-off, forgotten or 'lost' parts of themselves, as well as the corresponding repressed emotions. If these are transferred and projected onto the therapists, they can be interpreted. Making conscious and overt such projections is believed to induce new reflections and perspectives, enabling better interactions and communications within the family (Skynner 1976). Therapists also make use of 'counter-transference' feelings evoked in them, which contribute to an understanding of how individual family members, or the family as a whole, get fixed in roles or positions that 'suit' them. One way of thinking about this is to imagine an iceberg with all the conscious thoughts, memories and feelings being above the water. Analytical ideas seek to put into accessible form all those experiences below the waterline.

The structural approach

The *structural approach* (Minuchin 1974, Minuchin and Fishman 1981) largely replaced, or perhaps more accurately eclipsed, analytical ideas in the late 1960s and early 1970s, because of course, old ideas are often to be found embedded within

Noticing and using transference

Psychoanalytic family therapy is hardly practised these days. Yet, some of the ideas can be helpful in primary care settings. Practitioners will often develop strong counter-transferences to specific patients. Examining these evoked feelings, whether positive or negative, and reflecting on how they had arisen, can be of considerable 'diagnostic' value (Balint 1957). Some patients present themselves in such a deprived state that it is impossible not to feel moved and spring into action to 'help'. Pausing and reflecting before doing so can be useful when trying to understand what the patient, couple or family are consciously or unconsciously trying to make you do.

the new and often to their benefit. So, away with the obsession with the past and transference! Instead, this approach focuses on understanding and changing problematic family 'structures' (interaction and communication patterns) in the 'here and now'. Examples of these are 'dysfunctional' hierarchies between the generations, or 'inadequate' boundaries between parents and their children. Structural therapists attempt to actively change these, with the aim of making the family structure more 'normal'. This approach does, of course, have some problems, as the notions of 'normal' and 'dysfunctional' can feel a little like some form of social engineering, particularly if the clinicians believe that their view of what is normal is superior or 'true' or 'right'. Of course the idea that we do not find ourselves judging another's behaviour against our own ideas of behaviour is a nonsense. We do. Yet a way out of this potential problem is for clinicians to elicit from each family member what *they* themselves regard as 'better' ways of being with one another. The clinician's stance is then not moralistic or prescriptive, but facilitative in assisting the family to achieve their goals. This can best be done by direct observation of couple and family interactions in the consulting room or, better still, in the home. Seeing 'live', as it were, what goes on, helps the clinician to draw attention to how family members get into difficult – and familiar – impasses.

Transference and you – making the connection

- Think of a patient, couple or family you have seen recently and who has evoked some surprisingly strong feelings in you, such as a fierce urge to be extra helpful, or a strong feeling of disgust or even hatred.
- Think what it was that provoked this feeling. Was it something 'in' the patient?
- Search your mind whether it resonates with some of your own life situation or past experiences.
- Try doing your own family tree and see if there are any links (see Chapter 5).
- Discuss this with a colleague you trust.

Furthermore, it allows various interventions, such as commenting on and then challenging directly any absent or rigid boundaries. 'Homework' tasks can be designed to restore such boundaries and, if required, re-establish some family hierarchies.

Next please . . .

Mrs E comes repeatedly, often with her husband, to discuss her ambivalence about taking HRT, which she stops and starts every six or eight weeks. She makes her GP feel bewildered, often furious and like a mother who just can't treat her adolescent daughter right. Circular questions have not been helpful, the other partners have tried being bossy and the consultant gynaecologist says she has nothing more to say on the subject. Saying to them both: 'I have noticed over the years that sometimes people have relationships with their doctors and medication that are like the relationships they had with one of their parents' produced an interesting response. Mrs E's husband said that her mother had never listened to her and always made decisions for her, which made her feel put down. Mrs E said that she thought it was important that she had control of her HRT but that her mother was irrelevant to this. So the GP was able to decide just to sit it out, and be consistent and occasionally firm – perhaps as firm as parents of adolescents need to be.

The move to concentrate on the 'here and now' is a profound shift in ways of thinking and behaving with patients. There is a widespread belief in many modern Western cultures that 'if only you had time to hear about all the details of my upbringing . . . then you would understand . . . and then you could make it better for me'. In a curious way, just as popular culture was getting heavily into 'upbringing determines adult behaviour' so this branch of family therapy (and others to come) was saying 'maybe, maybe not, but let's concentrate on what you are doing now and how we might change the steps'.

Next please . . .

Ms H, the practice nurse, visited Mrs W twice weekly to dress a post-operative wound. She noticed that the person with most authority in the family was the youngest child, Kate. Kate tried to boss Ms H around the moment she came into the house. 'You are late, my mum has been waiting for you.' Her father, Mr W, would reply (with a big smile): 'Kate, don't be so cheeky!' Kate just replied: 'Shut up!' and Mr W would then turn to the practice nurse, shrugging his shoulders, saying weakly: 'She thinks she is the boss.' Mr W then spoke about their teenage children: 'She is just copying them . . . they do what they want.' Mrs W turned to her husband: 'You are never here and that's why they run riot!' Ms H observed all this and resisted the temptation to get involved. What should she have done? Was this an opportunity to intervene? Had she been a structural therapist, she might be tempted to work with this 'action'. She might have asked each parent whether they were 'happy' with how things were going in the family and, if they weren't, what specifically they might want to change. Did they like their daughter running the show, for example?

The structural approach deliberately focuses on what is going on between people, whether in the home or in the consulting room. Sometimes it is possible to get a spontaneous glimpse of specific couple or family issues. On other occasions the clinician can actively encourage partners or other family members to 'enact' problematic issues, whether arguments about in-laws, money or how to punish a naughty child.

Observing, challenging, enacting

Clinicians can experiment with the following model:

'I notice you all argue very loudly ... I have now witnessed how things escalate. I do not need to see nor hear any more. Let me ask each of you: Is that the way you want it?' [Patients usually respond that they do not want more arguments.] 'So, if you don't want it that way, how would you like it to be?' [This allows each family member to present a 'vision' of how they would like things to be.] 'What could each of you do or say now, so that you have a different outcome, the outcome you both want?'

This sequence is designed to get the 'combatants' to pause for reflection and to find alternative ways of resolving conflictual issues. It can be used in many circumstances:

- 'I notice that when I ask you a question your father often helps you with the reply, is that how you want it?'
- 'I notice that since John's heart attack, you have got very good at anticipating all his needs and doing things for him. Is that the way both of you want it?'

Next please ...

A couple came to see their GP with their 18-month-old boy who was keeping them awake every night with constant demands for bottles of milk and by repeatedly waking up. They wanted advice on what to do about it. The GP asked about sleeping patterns in the house in general and rapidly established that they had a 5-year-old daughter who was still sleeping in their bed, in between them. She had apparently been there since birth. The clinician, who does not like his own children sleeping in the bed with him, managed NOT to say 'Are you crazy?!' but instead asked more playfully: 'How on earth did you manage to conceive the second one then?!' After some genuine laughter, he discovered that the grandparents had had the daughter over the weekend on that single occasion. His next remark was simple and useful: 'Is this the way you want it to be?' It became clear that the parents were agreed that they did not want it to be like that. Exploration of boundaries and stumbling-blocks on their way to insisting on some new night-time routines was helpful. With the support of the health visitor and over a couple of weeks the parents negotiated the move out of their bed for the elder child and then a sleep programme for the younger one. They succeeded and were pleased with their success.

Strategic family therapy

Another school of systemic practice developing in the late 1960s was *strategic family therapy* (Haley 1963, Watzlawick *et al.* 1974), which aimed to deliver interventions, or 'strategies', to fit the presenting problems. One of the underlying assumptions of the approach is that the illness – or problem – is being maintained by the apparent 'solution', namely the very behaviours that seek to suppress the presenting problem. For example, Mrs C, suffering from depression and low self-esteem, elicits her husband's overprotectiveness. This seemingly appropriate 'solution' can become a problem in its own right as it may contribute to the perpetuation of the problem. Strategic therapists use the technique of 'reframing': the problem is put into a different meaning-frame which introduces a new perspective. For example, Mrs C's 'problem' can be reframed as her being very competent in making her husband feel useful, being a much needed carer, so much so that he does not have to face his own personal issues.

Tasks

Some strategic techniques can be used in primary care. A strategic prescription in Mrs C's family would consist of asking the husband to respond to his wife's seeming neediness only on *even* days of the week, and to be deliberately non-helpful on the *uneven* days. This 'task' would have to be carried out over a period of a fortnight, with each partner making their own observations and notes separately. The results can then be discussed during the next consultation. The aim of this intervention is not only for an experimental undoing of a familiar pattern, but also for each partner to become observers to their own interactions. This allows them to have different views of themselves, leading to different actions.

Strategic approaches rely quite heavily on the power of the therapist or team to deliver the strategy and encourage clients to 'try it out'. Sometimes the trust that is placed in primary care clinicians allows for a similar prescription. At other times it can feel difficult to deliver such strategies because they feel so different to the way we usually work. However, you may find various more gentle prescriptions helpful.

> *'Perhaps next time you are on the verge of disagreeing with her again, you might like to try the reverse. Do an experiment and agree fully and unreservedly. If she tries to challenge you, refuse to take the bait, trying to be as genuine as you can. In fact explore whether you could not just agree, but also convince yourself that nothing will be gained for being 'right' – therefore just go along with what she thinks is right. Under no circumstances tell her that your agreement is only strategic – you yourself need to be determined that there is no point about arguing who is right – just behave as if she is. Let me know next time how it went.'*

The Milan systemic approach

Another school of thought, the early *Milan systemic approach* (Selvini Palazzoli *et al.* 1978), focused on family patterns that have evolved over generations and are so powerful that they organise family life in the present. Typical examples are young adults, often presenting with psychotic disorders or 'bizarre' behaviours, who seem to get caught up between their warring parents who continuously disqualify one another. Such disqualifications are often linked to socially 'inherited' interaction styles from the respective families of origin. A disqualification is a communication affirmed at one level whilst being disconfirmed at another: 'Of course, you must do what you think is right', said in a very angry tone of voice, can be a first step in an interaction of mutual disqualification. If a family member is disqualifying their own and others' messages, it will be easy for everybody else to reciprocate. Often the only response to messages that conflict on different levels is an escalation of more messages that conflict on different levels (Haley 1963). Thus a vicious circle of mutual disqualification evolves, which, once established, is hard to stop. Children and young persons presenting with 'bizarre' or psychotic behaviours can seem like the victims of such communication styles.

Families with such complex intra-familial interaction styles also have a tendency to disqualify therapists. They are notoriously difficult to help and the Milan team specialised in the treatment of these seemingly intractable families. In fact, the team designed interventions which took into account the anticipated attempts of the family to disqualify the therapy. The resulting 'counter-paradoxes' prescribed by the team were aimed at recommending 'no change', in the hope that the family would resist this command and do the opposite, namely change – if only to defeat the therapist(s)! Paradoxical prescriptions were fashionable in the 1980s but are rarely used nowadays (see Chapter 10). However, what has survived from the early Milan approach is a particular style of interviewing that is in itself an intervention: circular and reflexive questioning (Selvini Palazzoli *et al.* 1980). This technique is described in considerable detail in Chapter 4.

In the early 1980s the original Milan team divided into two groups. One team pursued their interests in unravelling the 'games' of psychotic and anorectic families (Selvini Palazzoli *et al.* 1989). They became preoccupied with designing an 'invariate' prescription, which included secret pacts with the therapist and mysterious parental disappearance acts. The aim of this rather dramatic approach was to disrupt chronic family organisation, and the rather hypnotic techniques seemed to work for some families but not for others (see Chapter 10). The other half of the original Milan team (Boscolo *et al.* 1987), now called Milan Associates, went in the opposite direction, away from any prescriptiveness. Their commitment to 'positive connotation' has produced a non-blaming approach which is still embraced by many systemic practitioners: the actions of all family members are seen primarily as the best everyone could do under the circumstances; even if the outcomes of family members' actions were seemingly negative, the intentions are viewed as positive.

The clinician as observer or participant?

First-order cybernetics conceptualised families and other social systems as being self-regulatory, describing them in terms of their functioning, their rules and feedback processes. The clinicians saw themselves as being outside observers. The term second-order cybernetics was introduced to depict the shift of focus from an 'objective' therapist observing an 'object', such as a family. Instead the emphasis was moved onto the interaction between the observing and the observed systems, with the therapist being viewed as a collaborative explorer. Postmodern therapists, influenced by this new epistemology, continuously reflect on their own expectations, beliefs and perceptions, attempting to co-create with their clients and families some new ways of being and seeing.

Positive connotation

This is a reframing technique: the clinician views and feeds back to the family and its individual members positive reasons for all their behaviours and actions. It is based on an
assumption – or indeed a deliberate therapeutic 'prejudice' – that even when the outcome
is not good, people do nevertheless have good intentions and common goals – above all
to preserve the cohesion of the family group (Selvini Palazzoli *et al.* 1978). This positive
stance is very reassuring to most patients and families – at least for a while. It is non-
blaming. Searching for what is positive does not come easy for professionals who have
been trained to specialise in looking for pathology. Finding positive frames for seemingly
dysfunctional behaviour or symptoms is therefore a challenge. Those of you who are
involved in appraising other clinicians may like to speculate about whether you use the
same techniques with patients and with colleagues. If it is possible to 'frame' or positively
connote a colleague's behaviour, then might it be possible to find such a frame for a
patient's behaviour? Remember that positive connotation is not the same as condoning
behaviour, and it is still quite possible to notice parts of behaviour that are more
problematic, but many find change easier if there is some joint sense that at least in places
they are trying their hardest.

The Milan Associates and their followers, inspired by the writings of physicists,
neuroscientists and philosophers (Von Foerster and Zopf 1962, Maturana and Varela
1980), in the 1980s started examining the position of the therapist as being allegedly
a neutral observer of the family system. They found that therapists are actively
involved in constructing what is being observed. This realisation paralleled a much
wider postulate in the philosophy of science that scientists were not neutral and
objective either, but actively influenced the very experiments they thought they were
just observing (for those with an interest in these esoteric ideas: this was one of
the roots of postmodernism). Involving the patient in this process leads to a joint
'co-construction' of the therapeutic agenda. Both in therapy and in family life,
interactions and their meanings are co-constructed over time.

The social constructionist approach

The most recent phase of systemic therapy has been influenced by the *social constructionist approach*. This is based on the awareness that the 'reality' therapists
observe is 'invented', with perceptions being shaped by the therapists' own cultures,
their implicit assumptions and beliefs and the language they use to describe things.
Foucault's view that each culture has dominant narratives and discourses (Foucault
1975) has influenced many systemic practitioners and has led to an examination of
how language shapes problem perceptions and definitions (Goolishian and Anderson
1987). The notion of the 'problem-determined' system (Anderson *et al.* 1986) refers
to how interactions between clinicians and clients or families are programmed by the
built-in assumptions inherent in the traditional clinical discourses employed to discuss

experiences and relationships. As long as therapeutic encounters focus on clients' experiences as evidence of illness or pathology, then they remain trapped in pathology frames. They and their clinicians are able to make sense of their experiences within that framework. However, if the narratives in which clients 'story' their experience – or have their experience 'storied' by others – do not fit these experiences, then significant aspects of their lived experience will contradict the dominant narrative (White and Epston 1990) and be experienced as problematic.

Narrative-based primary care practitioners see their main task as helping the patient to develop a new story (Hurwitz 2000, Launer 2002). Patients' initial narratives about the illness or problem are often fragmented, complicated and confused. The clinician's narrative may be so dominant that it takes over the consultation, instead of developing a shared new narrative that is an improvement on the opening one. Anderson *et al.* (1986) also developed ideas of the problem dis-solving system of care. It is chilling to think that the systems of care we set up, for instance to make back pain better, may dissolve the problem by having long waiting times which cause people to develop unhelpful beliefs and behaviour patterns around their pain. It is interesting to reflect how often this happens in primary care.

Systemic narrative therapy

Systemic narrative therapy aims to enable clients and families to generate and evolve new stories and ways of interpreting past and present events to make sense of their experiences. Therapy is seen as a mutually validating conversation, between patient and clinician, from which change can occur. They 'co-evolve' or 'co-construct' new ways of describing their own issues and family or couple dynamics, so that these no longer need to be viewed or experienced as problematic. Clinicians practising in this way tend to describe themselves as being even-handed and realistic about the possibility of change, with no wish to impose their own ideas, being alert to openings as well as remaining curious about their own position in the observed system, taking non-judgemental and multipositional stances (Jones 1993). Quite a task!

Central to this approach is the process of reflection which is seen – as it is in other approaches – as necessary to promote change. The 'reflecting team' (Andersen 1987) is one of the major innovations in recent years. No longer are there 'secret' discussions between clinician and team members behind a one-way screen; these now take place openly in front of the family. The implied sharing of the clinicians' thinking with clients involves the latter in a process of reflection rather than imposing interventions on them.

Another useful approach emerging from narrative therapies is the *'externalisation of problems'*, which is both an orientation as well as a technique used by narrative therapists (White 1997). This encourages families to personify the problem they experience as oppressive so that the problem becomes a separate entity external to the person (White and Epston 1990). For example, in work with encopretic children, the child is asked to think of the soiling as his enemy who is given the name 'sneaky pooh'. This enemy needs to be defeated at all costs (White 1989). The help of the family is enlisted to devise strategies to trick this imaginary monster. Soon everyone joins forces to outwit sneaky pooh, who now becomes enemy number one for the whole family. A number of ingenious steps are employed to defeat 'the enemy' involving all family members in playful interactions. This approach has been applied to a whole range of symptoms and conditions, from anorexia to depression and schizophrenia.

Reflecting teams

This approach was originally pioneered in primary care settings in Norway (Andersen 1987). Patients found this a very empowering experience – to listen to the clinical discussion the team had about them. In this way they became active participants in, rather than passive recipients of, the clinicians' thoughts and formulations. Just consider this:

- What would happen if your most problematic patient was a fly on the wall in your weekly practice meeting?
- Would they be shocked, amused, delighted?
- What might your patient's reflections on your reflections be?
- Supposing the family reflected back on what you thought about them.

What this approach does, among many things, is to invite us to think more carefully about how we construct stories about our patients. It may be hard sometimes not to want to leave a room and simply say: 'It is not surprising he is so odd – just look at his mother!' And sometimes, of course, clinicians need somewhere to be 'unprofessional'. However, the key is in detecting when such unhelpful formulations start to permeate the way one is thinking about a patient 'in the room'. After all, this is only one hypothesis about what may be happening and not one that would help the patient find a more useful frame for change.

Next please . . .

Mrs F presented to her GP with incapacitating panic attacks associated with episodes of apparent paralysis. One of the many small things that helped was to start to externalise the panic attacks and name them as a thing separate from her. They became a monster with a name and separate from her sense of who she was. One of the early tasks was to say 'hello' to the monster, to look it in the eye and to discover that it could do her no harm. She chose a small gong to represent the monster and still carries it in her bag. There have been plenty of struggles with somatic complaints since then but that particular monster holds little fear.

Next please . . .

Mr C came to see the nurse practitioner with low mood. The practitioner started to ask some slightly different questions:

- *'What shall we call this set of feelings that has such influence and power over your life right now?'*
- *'When does Sadness seem to be able to ruin your life the most?'*
- *'Are there any occasions when you reduce the ability of Sadness to muck up your day?'*
- *'What things do you have to do so that Sadness does not get such a look in?'*
- *'Now how was it that yesterday Sadness was on the run?'*
- *'Are you aware of anything you do that aids and strengthens Sadness?'*
- *'Does anyone else have a major positive or negative affect on how Sadness operates in your life?'*

Mr C became more interested in his relationship with Sadness and saw himself as separate from it and slightly more able to think of ways he could start to reduce its influence on his life.

Solution-focused therapy

Brief solution-focused therapy (de Shazer 1982) emphasises the competencies of families and individuals. It deliberately does not focus at all on the 'problem-saturated' ways of talking and instead examines carefully the patterns of previous attempted solutions. The approach is based on the observation that symptoms and problems have a tendency to fluctuate. A depressed person, for example, is sometimes more and sometimes less depressed. Focusing on the times when they are less depressed are the exceptions on which therapeutic strategies are built. These exceptions form the basis of the solution. If clients are encouraged to amplify the 'solution' patterns of behaviours, then the problem patterns can be driven into the background.

One of the most helpful ideas from this field is the idea of moving from problem-saturated conversations to more solution-orientated conversations. How often have you felt exhausted after listening to a well-known patient spend 12 minutes recounting the complexity and depth of their problems? Now, of course, it is respectful and important to 'hear' these problems. But when you are hearing the fifth rendition of these problems in as many weeks, it can become not only exhausting for you and the patient but also unhelpful. It is as if you are both stuck in a quagmire of problems where there is no hope. However, just beyond this problem-saturated bog you could discover that the patient still manages to visit an elderly relative who has Alzheimer's, is still managing to make model airplanes, actually runs the karaoke session in the local pub.

Searching for these 'exceptions to the rule' – as solution-focused therapists put it – or for 'news of difference' as Bateson (1972) might have put it – is more or less the same for our purposes, to develop a solution-orientated conversation'.

'Next time you come I would like you to tell me one thing about your day that has been positive' or *'I am interested in how you have still managed to visit Mrs Blain despite all your troubles.'*

A solution-orientated conversation, is, if nothing else, a refreshing change for you both! Primary care, indeed health care settings in general, invite the telling of problems and all the good bits get left out. They are left at home, left in the unexplored context of people's lives. But it is in the 'good bits' that we are likely to find the strengths, resources and energies to effect the change that is needed. Solution-focused practitioners are good at harnessing these bits and they have a good place, at times, in primary care.

The psycho-educational approach

Another family therapy model that has been influential over the years, particularly since it has a strong evidence base, is the *psycho-educational approach* (Leff *et al.* 1982, Anderson 1983). This contains behavioural elements but also draws on structural techniques. The model is based on the findings that schizophrenics who return to live with a family whose attitudes towards the ill person are critical or emotionally over-involved (high EE = high expressed emotion) are significantly more likely to relapse in the nine months following discharge from hospital than those patients who return to low EE families. Consequently, the aim of therapy is

The miracle question

The miracle question (Berg 1991) has become one of the trademarks of the solution-focused approach. There are many versions and it can be used with some success in primary care situations. The clinician may say:

> Now just for a moment imagine that tonight when you were asleep a miracle happened. Somehow everything in your life was suddenly how you wanted it to be. It was as if a fairy godmother had come and waved a magic wand over your life. BUT you were asleep at the time. So when you woke up you did not at first realise that the miracle had happened, that everything was how you always wanted it to be. Then you started to notice things were different. What did you notice? Can you try and describe for me what it would look like, feel like, be like if the miracle had happened?

Initially patients are inclined to say one of two things. Either they say 'It won't happen', to which the reply is, 'Well let's just imagine for a moment that it did', to try to push them towards some sense of what they want and to invite them to look beyond the quagmire of problems for a moment. Or they start with global statements 'I would feel happy'. The clinician can then say: 'Great, and what would be happening, would you be alone or with someone, would you be living here or else where, what would you be doing?'

The purpose of the miracle question is to invite the patient to paint a concrete detailed and optimistic picture of a life where everything was going better for them. Sometimes the very act of trying to do this reveals how little of their time has been spent thinking about what it could be like. So much time has been spent in the problem-saturated quagmire. Simply inviting them to 'envision' a better place can then start to generate some energy for change.

The next task of course is to take from this larger picture small steps that might be already happening or small steps that might be taken in the direction of this better picture.

It is not always easy and takes practice to work this way. It lends itself well to the short consultation as you can ask the patient or patients to work on the miracle question at home, to bring back notes or more thoughts to paint in details on their own or better still in discussion with others: 'So what do you think should be part of the miracle picture?'

to reduce the emotional intensity as well as the degree of physical proximity. This is achieved by essentially using three separate therapeutic ingredients: educational sessions for the family about schizophrenia and the part the family can play in keeping the patient well; fortnightly relatives' groups to share experiences and solutions; and family sessions (Kuipers *et al.* 1992). It has been established that an intensely conflictual and overprotective, if not claustrophobic, family atmosphere is harmful to family members prone to psychotic breakdowns. Primary care clinicians can help to reduce the levels of expressed emotion in carers by means of psycho-education, by helping to reduce intra-family conflicts and by modifying the living circumstances of some of these families, such as housing.

This model has become influential in the development of services for patients with psychotic illness in the UK, with successful training programmes (Falloon

1988), such as the Meriden project in the West Midlands. There are many challenges for primary care clinicians in getting involved with supporting the families of those with psychotic symptoms and other severe mental illnesses. However, simply attempting to understand the impact of such illness and being aware of other family members seems the least we should be able to expect of generalist clinicians.

Future histories

Once upon a time, there were many different schools of systemic work, fiercely competing with one another, each claiming to have a 'better' model. Then the field started to grow up and things continued to change as systemic practitioners left behind their adolescent battles. In a more mature middle age, collaboration and integration of different systemic approaches and techniques are common. Practitioners have discovered that there are more similarities than differences between the various approaches. Moreover, we have also learned that different families and presentations require different therapeutic responses. However, what all systemic approaches have in common is a belief in interventive questioning, a conviction that asking questions stimulates reflection. Some therapists like to be more active, others sit back. A current development is the rediscovery of psychodynamic roots, back to where it all started, but with a new story emerging.

Beyond Balint

Involving the whole family in treatment is an obvious idea. Looking at physical or emotional symptoms in context makes sense when one remembers that most people are involved in relationships. Illness can affect relationships and, in turn, will be affected by the responses of key relatives. The family approach acknowledges that people have their own personal 'hi-stories' and problems and it therefore does not challenge the value of good individual consultation skills. Michael Balint's influential work (Balint 1957, Balint *et al.* 1993) has contributed to an understanding of how patients may communicate through their symptoms with their doctors. The family approach complements Balint's work by providing a practical way of managing patients and their problems, integrating physical, psychological and social approaches. Its emphasis is less on how to review or change the past, more on how to tackle the present and how to do things differently in the future. It therefore has the advantages of helping primary care workers to conceptualise their patients' problems in a fresh and useful way. It works very much in the 'here and now' and helps people to question their frameworks and change their perspectives. It encourages people not to get trapped by their past experiences, challenges their current thinking and gets them to experiment with new solutions. It stresses the importance of asking questions that enable patients to make sense of their symptoms and to change their outlook.

Questioning and reflecting on the agenda

4

This chapter covers:
- ○ Circular questions
- ○ Curiosity
- ○ Reflexivity

Questions are the very 'stuff' of primary care and of the clinical encounter. They are ultimately the way we – either as patient or as clinician – construct meaning in our lives. Patients come with questions – questions about their symptoms and problems: 'What is the matter with my head?' 'Why am I always so tired?' 'When will the pain stop?' 'Who can help me?' 'How can I feel better?' And they expect answers to these questions; at least they do some of the time, although probably much less often than their clinicians think they do. At the very least they expect to talk about the questions they bring. Clinicians also bring questions to the encounter. We know that there are usually no easy answers to be given, certainly not without further inquiry, and before coming up with any 'answers or prescriptions', we feel the need to find out more.

It is good clinical practice to start any inquiry by posing questions, in the hope that the answers will throw some light on the presenting problem or symptom(s). In the past clinicians have tended to have a rather simple view of questions and questioning. It has been viewed merely as the way of gaining information and facts. The task as a clinician in training is usually to memorise the 'right' list of questions in the 'right' order so that a 'proper history' of the complaint can be laid out. Who remembers writing 'poor historian' in the notes of patients who appeared not to be able to answer the comprehensive and linearly ordered questions of their interrogator?

A systemic approach to questions has more to say about the matter. This chapter will explore the idea that questions are not neutral or objective, but organised by context and feedback, as well as being subjective. Questions can be seen as interventions in the consultation, able to bring forth new ideas and perspectives, able to change understanding and meaning. Systemic practitioners also place questioning in a broader context. Questions can be asked not just of the person but of the symptom itself and of the wider system of which the patient and the symptom are part. Questions are a rich source of interest both for clinicians and, more importantly, for their patients.

Content and process

One way of thinking about many situations, including clinical encounters (but it is just as useful in committee meetings or any social interaction), is to divide the encounter into its content – the facts, bits of information, details of the story – and the process – the what is going on, how the story is being told, how you relate to it, what emotions are being expressed by them, by you, in the room. To use the analogy of the dance, which we have employed throughout this book, content pays attention to what each step looks like in detail but often fails to pay attention to the way the steps fit together; the *process* turns individual steps into an interactional dance.

This may sound obvious, but it is surprising how often, particularly when stuck for where to go next, we opt for a closed question that elicits more content rather than pause and reflection. What is the process?

This idea that more content will help is deeply ingrained in much professional training and can be hard to shake off or at least balance with an interest in process. The technique (Observing, challenging, enacting) described in the Fruit Box in the previous chapter (page 36) is used to comment directly on such processes. The 'inner consultation' (Neighbour 1987) is a useful framework for learning to pay attention to both process and content.

Questioning the symptom

In primary care the questions: What? Why? When? Who? How? guide the clinician to formulate ideas, possibly to make a diagnosis and to inform subsequent actions, including treatment options. This is the bedrock of the clinical method and a crucial skill which has served clinicians well over centuries. However, at times other sorts of questioning may be more useful. Systemic practitioners often find it useful to question the symptom – and not the patient. This can be done in a number of ways, even before the patient arrives in the room.

All questions about the symptom share a similar organising idea, namely that symptoms are not just 'out there' like objects attached to individuals. Instead, they are seen as being at least in part created in the space between people, not just inside individuals. They have an interactional dimension.

Take, for example, the symptom of a high temperature. Of course, no one doubts that infectious diseases produce fevers and that these may be experienced as high temperature. Whether this becomes a symptom or not is another matter. Is this a family that uses thermometers? Is it only a symptom if it is unexpected or noticed? Is it a symptom only because the patient's elder brother died after a high temperature was missed? Is it a symptom only in a culture that believes fevers to be bad and so need eradicating with fans and antipyretics? Does high temperature mean temperature above 39 degrees or high seriousness, something that emphasises the perceived illness of the child?

Some things become symptoms because the clinician is interested in them – the patient may not have seen them as symptoms at all. Others become symptoms because the client thinks they are when the clinicians may not! So one thing

Questioning the symptom – reflective practice

What is the symptom that the patient presents?

- What are its effects? What function might it serve?
- What is the context within which the symptom occurs? What is
- happening when the symptom is present?

Why is the symptom present?

- Why *now*? Why *this* symptom?

When is the symptom present?

- When did it start? When is it worse, when is it better?
- When is the symptom not present?

Who has the symptom?

- Who is around when the symptom happens? Who can make it better, who makes it worse?
- Who is affected by the symptom and in what way?

How does the symptom affect the family and how does the family (and others) affect the symptom?

---

clinicians may find useful before they barrage their patients with all sorts of questions, is to reflect and speculate about the role and 'life' of the symptom. In fact, some symptoms seem to have a life, if not a career, of their own. They change over time. They are constructed acutely when they first appear and they may change, or are 'differently storied', when they become chronic. The 'dance' around an acute symptom can be very different from the 'dance' around a chronic one. This can be explored by asking the following questions: 'When this first appeared in your lives what effects did it have? Have those changed over the time you have been living with this symptom?'

The posing of questions will focus a clinician's line of inquiry and help to formulate working hypotheses. Clinicians can ask and answer them 'in their heads', as it were, but they can also put some of these questions, or questions derived from them, to their patients. In this way the patients are involved in reflecting about the issues raised. Questions are so often more important than answers; the 'right' questions are often so much more powerful than the quick or 'right' answers. We are not suggesting that primary care workers should always reflect in such detail on each patient – time pressures will not permit this. However, when dealing with patients who present with time-consuming chronic problems, it may nevertheless be an economic way of generating new ideas.

Next please . . .

Mr W has suffered from chronic back pain for more than a year. Various physical investigations have not turned up any 'organic' causes for the pain. A substantial number of primary care workers have been hired – and fired – by Mr W, with plenty of frustration on all sides. Dr D is new to the health centre and she decides to take a different approach when Mr W makes an appointment to see her. Having read the extensive case notes she reflects about the 'story so far', prior to the consultation.

She asks a number of questions: what are the effects of Mr W's back problem on those living with him? Dr D speculates that Mr W might get a lot of sympathy, and he might get out of doing uncomfortable tasks or jobs at home. The bad back could have the 'function' of keeping the right distance between him and his wife. It might make her feel sorry – or angry. After reflecting on the possible 'spin-offs', Dr D then considered the negative effects of Mr W's chronic back problems on those near and dear. It would be quite possible to imagine that everyone at home was fed up with his continuous complaining – maybe the whole family needed to be rescued from the back pain, or the 'pain in the back'. Dr D then speculated about the why, the cause(s) of the back trouble. No identifiable organic pathology had been found – so did this mean it was 'all in the mind'? Dr D was too experienced to believe in simple explanations – probably there was some physical cause that accounted for why the pain was located in the back. Yet, the pain's persistence and severity almost certainly had something to do with how Mr W processed stress or pain.

One hypothesis Dr D entertained was that all stress converged on a locus minoris resistentiae, the spine, resulting in stress pain. If this hypothesis had some value, then it should be possible to speculate that, depending on stress levels, the pain level should fluctuate: when the pain started, when it is stronger or lesser – the time context – would need to be explored. Clues to possible answers might be provided by considering who was around during these pain fluctuations – and who had an effect on the pain, either for better or worse. How those near and dear responded to the back pain, and how the back pain responded to their reactions would also seem worth exploring.

After reflecting for a few minutes in this way, Dr D had plenty of ideas and hypotheses before Mr W entered the consulting room. She was very curious which of her hypotheses could be corroborated – and which refuted. Mr W was very pleasantly surprised that a doctor could be so interested in his pain and the family.

The importance of curiosity

One of the most important tools from the primary care survival kit is 'curiosity' (Cecchin 1987). As long as the clinician becomes or remains curious about the patient, the problem and the larger context, then there is hope – for both. A bored clinician tends to be a useless clinician. One of the functions of new approaches to the consultation is simply to help the clinician stay interested. It is not that all models and ideas are equally useful but many may have the simple function of encouraging the clinician to keep wondering about the lives and stories of their patients. The stance of curiosity is one where continously new perspectives on the patient's symptoms and predicament are generated, thus widening and changing the field of vision. The curious clinician will want to make the connections between

Curiosity

If you were to take only one word away from this book, then maybe it should be curiosity. It may have killed the cat, but because the cat had nine lives it experienced so much more! Health care professionals need a guiding word to keep them living their nine lives.

Curiosity guides making hypotheses and testing them out with questions. Of course, all clinicians need some 'solid ground' every now and then. So much of primary care is already uncertain. Don't you love that feeling when you arrive at solid ground – 'Hurrah, THIS is what is happening!' – and the patient usually likes it too. After all, coming to a clinician is in part about saying 'make it clear and certain'. But perhaps when the solid ground you seem to be on is not shared by the patient, or the problem does not resolve, or the feeling of joint arrival at certainty does not happen, then is the time to get out curiosity again. I wonder if .... Another way of thinking about this might be ...

otherwise unseen aspects of the patient's life and relationships, past or present, examining how the mind speaks for the body at one moment and how the body speaks for the mind at another (Elder 1996).

Good questions are characterised by their ability to open up new perspectives: they need to provide new information, not only for the clinician but, more importantly, for the patient. If a question triggers the patient to think thoughts that were previously unthinkable, then such a process of questioning leads patients to look at their problems from a different angle. This makes the finding of new ways forward – or even of solutions – possible.

As clinicians we are trained to formulate and entertain hypotheses which we use to corroborate or refute our investigations. Many of us feel the pressure of thinking that patients expect us to come up with quick answers. Time pressure may force a clinician to propose a premature 'solution' for a patient's predicament. Such solutions, ranging from 'try harder', to elaborate explanations as to why a patient 'is feeling like this', usually do not work terribly well although they may provide very temporary relief (albeit often only for the clinician!). However, sooner rather than later, the patient will return for further doses of advice until the clinician finally runs out of ideas and patience. Giving advice too quickly is the result of a mistaken belief that people are better off with answers. Yet, such 'answers' can deprive patients of the opportunity to question themselves, to reflect and to come up with answers for themselves.

Here is an example. Sore throats are a common symptom in general practice and are often caused by viruses or bacteria. They are usually self-limiting and of brief duration. Information of this sort, perhaps backed up with a leaflet, is often very useful. Patient and clinician are on shared firm ground and life can proceed. If the diagnosis is glandular fever then the ground can feel a little more shaky. To what extent should the clinician entertain the possibility of the illness lasting longer? Should this be mentioned and with what degree of authority or certainty? Do you mention the idea of more long-standing fatigue after glandular fever, or will this put the idea of 'ME' into the head of the patient? Questions can often come in useful here:

What have you heard about glandular fever? What is your current idea of how long it might last or what its consequences might be? Do you know whether anyone else in the family has a different view?

These sorts of preliminary questions can help the clinician to approach the task of arriving at a shared understanding of the consequences of the illness with more chance of success. Notice once again how all is not quite as it seems. It might appear that the traditional 10-minute appointment (and we know that some of you are consulting in even shorter time frames!) means that solutions have to be found in that time frame. Somehow the way we have chosen to organise time has had a direct influence on how we choose to behave in the consultation. But there are many assumptions driven by this temporal context. What about posing the following questions to the patient?

When you were coming down today did you have an idea about what you hoped might happen? What sort of solution did you think might appear at the end of our meeting?

Answers such as 'Well I knew that you can't solve this for me but I wanted to talk it through' can be extraordinarily liberating for the clinician if not the patient!

Feedback

Consulting with patients can be a dialogue, even a 'dance', but it should not be a set of parallel monologues, or the mutual exchange of unchanging facts! Examining feedback is an important activity that helps to decide what questions to ask next. The patient's responses both verbal and non-verbal prompt further questions which in turn lead to further responses, and so on. Asking questions and responding to answers is an interactive approach and as such is bound to produce feedback. This feedback can be divided into two types: content and process.

Content feedback

What patients actually say is of course very important information and needs to be listened to. It will help the clinician to confirm or discard a working hypothesis. It may open up the possibility of a new track and help to create different hypotheses that are based on the immediate feedback received from the patient. Together, patient and clinician can then explore new avenues. Early in their career, clinicians are often very interested in content. There is a widespread belief that 'If only we had all the details, then we would be able to reveal the mystery, make sense of it, explain what is happening.' This belief drives the desire for more closed questions, more diagnostic tests, more information. There are times when this is very important and equally there are times when all this quest does is move you further from understanding the dance, the pattern, relationship between people, symptoms and illnesses. Too many trees and no chance to see the pattern of the whole forest! This is where attention to process feedback is useful.

Process feedback

How patients respond gives important clues and the clinician in turn needs to respond to these. Hesitation, anger or reluctance to answer a specific question can indicate that the question has touched upon a sensitive area, which may require delicate exploration. Such responses can also be taken to mean that the issues raised are painful, maybe threatening, or simply irrelevant. Being at the receiving end of some intense process feedback from the patient can pose problems for clinicians. How should they deal with the patient's apparent resistance to answer certain questions or cover specific issues?

There are a number of different options. For example, the clinician could note (mentally) the patient's reluctance to answer, but stop pursuing this particular topic any further and think about when to take it up later. Careful thought about 'Why is it difficult to challenge this now?' can be revealing about underlying clinician, patient, illness and family processes. Alternatively, the clinician could decide to 'go for it' and say: 'That seems to be an uncomfortable question. Do you think it would help to talk about this now?' or 'Would you mind if I ask you some difficult or personal questions?'

Which of these two different options the clinician chooses will depend on a variety of factors: how well they know the patient; how comfortable they feel with handling any possible emotional outbursts; how fragile the patient appears; how much time is available, and so on. In the context of a good and trusting relationship, which may have evolved over considerable time, it may be best to use process feedback by taking up immediately areas of discomfort as they arise ('You look sad when we talk about your father. What is that about?'). However, time constraints may at times force the clinician to note a potential can of worms one day, but delay opening it until a later consultation when there is more time and space to tackle some of the issues.

Who answers questions can reveal a lot about family processes. Do husbands answer for their wives or wives talk over their husbands? Does one person start a sentence and another finish it? Does everyone talk at once? Below is a case example where mother speaks for her child. Questions can help to unpick the process observed in the room.

There are systemic clinicians who believe that the process of asking questions is sufficient to bring about change. Whatever the truth or otherwise of this belief, if the clinician *only* asks questions then some patients may start questioning the interviewer ('Why do you keep asking questions?' 'Why do you ask *me* that question – couldn't you ask my husband?' 'I want to know what *you* think, doctor'). In such circumstances it is important *not* to get into a confrontation with the patient, but take a one-down position by simply stating: 'It's the way I find most useful' or 'I just wanted to understand more, but if it is uncomfortable for you to answer all these questions I shall of course stop' (this often results in the patient giving explicit permission for the clinician to continue) or 'You are quite right, I should ask your husband, but he is not here at the moment. Do you mind therefore if I ask you now what he might say if he was here? You do not have to answer this if you don't want to or if you find it too difficult'.

Next please . . .

Emma (15¾) came with her mother to get a repeat prescription of the oral contraceptive pill for her painful periods. She had had genital warts treated by the practice nurse in the last year. With every question she looked to her mother for the first answer before joining in herself. She couldn't remember the name of the tablets she was taking. Both of them said that it was the other person's idea that they were both there. It seemed that she was entering the adult world of women with little sense of having control over her life, perhaps having been shamed by having genital warts. Here are some moderately 'subversive' questions:

- *'When you are 16 and you have a legal right to come and see me on your own, what would you have to do or think about before coming to the appointment?'*
- *'When your daughter is 16 and able to do things like sign consent forms for operations, how will your role as a mother be different?'*
- *'Learning to do all your own worrying and caring for yourself can take a while. How old would you like to be when you can do all these things for yourself?'*
- *'How old do you think your mum thinks you are – 8, 16 or 23?'*
- *'Tell me what would have to be different for your mum and you to agree on the age at which you are self-sufficient enough?'*
- *'What would your dad's view of this be?'*
- *'If your dad were here today would you be more or less likely to speak up?'*

The power of questions

Patients and families who consult their clinicians present what one might call 'stories' of their problems. There are myriad ways stories are presented, and

Illness stories

Stories are a way of thinking about clinical encounters as well as about patients' lives. They are mentioned throughout this book and a great deal has been written about them by other practitioners. For example, Arthur Kleinman writes about the particular ways clinicians might understand the illness narratives of patients (Kleinman 1988). He asserts that we have to try and understand the meaning of illness for each and every particular patient and it is only in attempting to do so that we can begin to help them with the illness, not the disease. Kleinman's book *Illness Narratives*, which he describes elsewhere as 'a populist account' (Kleinman 1995), is a first-rate introduction to the world of chronic illness, full of useful insights and thoughts about how to wrest healing from its technocratic tendencies and reposition it in human relationships.

There is a rich vein of literature with people writing about their own illness stories. One of the foremost authors is Arthur Frank, an anthropologist who developed cancer. In his book *The Wounded Storyteller* (Frank 1995), he succeeds in expanding the understanding of illness story types. He identifies three main categories: (1) The *restitution story* is much loved by patients and their clinicians: 'I was well, I got ill, heroic or mundane treatments were administered, I got better'. (2) The *chaos story* has no beginnings, middles or ends, only threads and confusion: 'Chaos stories are sucked into the undertow of illness and the disasters that attend it'. (3) In the *quest story*, patients 'meet suffering head-on; they accept illness and seek to use it'. Here the ill person believes there is something to be gained through the experience, including being able to tell the story. Frank speculates that much suffering is generated by the attempt by patients and practitioners to squeeze experience into stories that don't fit (Frank 1995).

experienced by patients. Here are a couple of common patterns: the practised story or routine, told as if it was true, written in stone, with people, events and problems welded together ('He is like that because he had a violent father and has not learned to handle his emotions'). Alternatively the story may be presented as an apparently random collection of persons and circumstances – disconnected, disjointed, seemingly arbitrary. Questioning these stories, which are often based on more or less fixed beliefs, is a way of getting such stories retold, thereby examining some of the implicit 'truths', beliefs and myths that helped to create and maintain them. Specific questions may allow the family to reflect about their life or problem stories, helping them to reinterpret these and discovering new solutions.

The process of questioning can be powerful if it aims to make the patient or family look at themselves in a new light. Patients are encouraged to view other people in relation to themselves as well as speculating how, in their view, others see them. In this way patients perceive themselves and their relationships through the eyes of other people and compare this with their own perceptions. This can help to make new connections between past, present and future; between symptoms and relationship issues; between assumptions and openly held opinions. It also allows patients to connect the present with future visions and actions.

Understanding the types of questions to use

Circular and reflexive questioning (Selvini Palazzoli *et al.* 1980) is an elegant technique which enables systemic clinicians to become curious inquirers who solicit information about the individual and other family members' beliefs and perceptions regarding relationships. By responding to the feedback provided, the clinician enacts 'circularity', basing the next question on the previous answer. The process of asking such reflexive questions gets individuals and families involved in writing or rewriting their stories: disjointed and random events become connected, fixed scripts start crumbling with new connections being made. Circular and reflexive questions are constructed by the clinician based on the initial information provided by the patient: linking questions to hypotheses creates a purposeful and coherent interviewing pattern where further questions are based on forthcoming answers which in turn inform further questions.

Reflexive and circular questions can be asked with just one person present, though they can be more powerful if other family members are present. Eliciting such information in the presence of family members and asking them to comment and reflect on the answers given by the various individuals, creates an infinite set of feedback loops which themselves change the fabric of family interactions. Each person could be asked the same question in turn, noting if not commenting on the different answers elicited. Triadic questions are particularly useful in that each person is asked to comment on the thoughts, behaviour and relationships of the other members of the family. A family member engaged in such a conversation has the opportunity to be an observer of others' perceptions about him rather than being involved in the action. So a different, more reflective sort of thinking is possible.

Below is a list of possible questions. These could never all be asked in the course of just one single consultation, of course. But remember that primary care workers have usually time on their side; they have many of their patients 'for life'. It does not all need to be fixed in the one session! Moreover, some of these questions may be entirely inappropriate for certain patients.

Examples of reflexive and circular questions

Problem/symptom questions

These aim to define the history of the problem or symptom, the contexts within which it occurs and the different responses to it.

- Who noticed your problem/symptom first? Who second? Who last?
- What is your explanation for the symptom/problem?
- What is your spouse's/father's/mother's explanation as to why you are having this problem? Do you agree with his/her view?
- What do you think made him/her form this opinion?
- If you wanted to change his/her mind about their view of your problem, how would you go about it?
- Who does what in response to the symptom?
- How does the problem affect your spouse/father/mother/children?
- When you're depressed/have pain, who responds to it first? What does s/he say or do? What happens next? How do you respond to his/her response? What happens then? And what is your response to that?
- Is there anybody who thinks that your problem is not 'real'? Or someone who believes that you are not ill, but just awkward? What is your response to that? What types of conversation between you and X does that produce?
- How come that X has this opinion? Do you think that X thinks that you could act differently?
- How do you know this? How good are you at working out what X or Y really thinks about your problem?
- What else might X or Y think or feel that they do not let you know about? How might they talk about your problem in your absence?
- What would you have to do to find out?
- If you did, what sorts of response might you get?

Solution-focused questions

These aim to identify current exceptions to the symptomatic behaviours and to highlight solutions already employed by the patient.

- I am interested in when the symptom does not happen. When are the times it happens less?
- How are you feeling and what are you doing when you don't have your irritable bowel pain?
- Tell me about what is happening when this isn't such a problem for you?
- If your daughter were here what would she have to say about times when things have been better?

Practice suggestion

Copy five different questions per week, put them on a memo pad in your consulting room. Try these questions out on 10 consecutive patients and record their responses.

- Looking back over the past few days, have there been times when you have been free of the problem or symptom? How do you account for that?
- If on a scale from 0 to 10, where 10 stands for your pain being unbearable and 0 for no pain, where do you think your husband would score you at present? Where would you score yourself? Was there a time during the past few days when it was less? What happened then? If you could do more of what happened then, is there a chance that the pain might more often be lower?
- Can you remember a time when you could have given into the problem, but you didn't? What happened then?
- If I was able to wave a magic wand and the problem disappeared, what would your life be like? What would be the first sign that you were overcoming the problem? How will you know when things begin to change?
- On a scale of 1 to 10, where would you place your father's depression now? Would he place it there, too? If not, why not?
- If you are one step up the scale what would be different? What else?

Help questions

These aim to clarify who wants help for what, as well as the implications of seeking and receiving help.

- Who in your family wants help most/who wants it least?
- What is your explanation for these differences?
- Who is most/least distressed about your problem?
- How did you decide that you should come and get some help?
- How did you discuss this and with whom? What were the sorts of responses?
- What would have happened if you had decided not to consult me?
- Does coming here for help make it easier or more difficult to discuss these things with him/her?
- Supposing you weren't coming here for help, how would you deal with this problem?
- What does s/he really think about you coming here for help? What do you think s/he imagines goes on here?
- Who'd be most/least in favour of you coping on your own rather than going for help?
- What do you think are the consequences if nothing is found which will help the problem? What will be the effects on you, on your partner/parent/child?

Change questions

These aim to explore the implications and consequences of change.

- I am going to ask you a question to which the answer is probably very obvious: How would you know you're getting better?
- What sort of observations would you make? What would be different?
- How would anybody else know?
- Supposing you did not tell anybody that your problem had got better, would X or Y notice anyway? What other signs would X or Y observe that might make them think that you were getting better?
- How would your partner/mother/child notice that you were getting better?
- How would your relationship with X or Y be affected if your problem got
- better? What would be the advantages? I know, it may seem a strange question, but are there any disadvantages in getting better?
- Supposing there were some disadvantages, and you decided that there might be something in it to keep the symptoms – would you be able to consciously produce them? What would you have to do? How would you go about doing this?
- What would X, Y, Z's response be if s/he knew?
- Supposing there was no change in your symptoms for another few months – which relationship would suffer most?

Relationship questions

These aim to examine communication and interaction patterns.

- How do you see the relationship between your brother and your mother?
- How do you think your father sees his relationship with you?
- How would your mother describe the relationship between you and your father?
- Would this be different from how you see it – or how your father sees it?
- How do you explain the differences between how X and Y see this relationship?
- If your wife was sitting here and heard you say this, what might she say?
- And if she did, how would you respond? And what would be her reply?
- Who is the closest/most distant to your father/mother? Who second/third most?
- Who agrees with you that X is closest to Y? Is there anyone who might have a different view? What do you think that is based on?
- You said this is the way it is (e.g. your relationship with X). What would have to happen for this to be different?
- Was there ever any time when this was different?
- What were things like before and after illness (death, separation) struck?
- Who suffered most/least from X's illness/death/birth?
- Who can cheer up/depress X or Y most?
- When do you feel most like a daughter, when like a mother, when like a wife? How do you explain this? Who else can make you feel like that?
- Who is most/least upset when you do not get on with X?

Hypothetical questions

These aim to reflect on the implications of new scenarios and hypothetical situations.

*   If you weren't around how would your parents get along without you?
*   `If one child were to stay at home, who would it be?
*   If you had not been born, what would your parents' marriage be like?
*   If your wife got suddenly better, who would next be ill?
*   Supposing your partner didn't have any physical symptoms, which of the children would be closer to their father?
*   If your mother spoke now, what might she say? And how might your father respond to that? And how would you respond to that?
*   You have already got considerable experience with doctors and other primary care workers. What would I have to do to make this treatment a failure too?
*   Supposing your partner had been a fly on the wall throughout all our meetings. What would she think about it all? Would you agree with her observations? Why not?
*   Supposing you let your wife negotiate all the contact with your mother and she took the responsibility for that. How would that affect your symptoms?
*   Supposing you asked your son to leave and insisted that your husband spends more time with you. How would that affect your headaches?
*   If your mother were still alive today, what do you think her opinion would be about the problems you are having with the children?

'Wild' questions

These aim to search for specific areas of strengths or problematic situations, as well as aiming to cause some 'perturbations'.

*   If there was one thing that your dad would, in your view, feel proud about, to do with you (your mother/sister/wife), what might this be?
*   Which of your strengths can your wife/father not see?
*   When was the last time that you think your children saw you and your wife being really happy together?
*   Each family has an alcoholic – who is it in your family?
*   There is sexual abuse in many families. If there was some in your family, where might this have been?
*   What is the 'night life' of your family like?
*   Supposing we were to imagine your family in five years' time having successfully negotiated this difficult patch, where would you all be and what would you be doing? How would you like to be getting on?
*   Just imagine that you are now at the end of your life. What else would you like to have done? How might you, 30 years on, counsel yourself about the dilemmas you are now facing?

Miracles revisited

The 'miracle question' (Berg 1991) has already been described in the previous chapter. It gets around the conscious thought processes that sometimes get in the way of thinking of times when things are different, by the question being imaginary.

> *I would like to ask you an unusual sort of question. Is that OK? I would like you to imagine that while you are asleep a miracle happens and the miracle is that you wake up in the morning able to cope with all the things that are difficult for you now. Because you are asleep you don't know this miracle has happened. What do you notice first? Who is the first person to notice that you are behaving differently? How long would it take for them to notice?*

Gradually the 'miracle' day gets elaborated on and generally surprises both clinician and patient. 'If tomorrow you chose to do one of the things you have talked about in your miracle day which thing will you choose? Is there another thing you will choose?' This question can be asked sensitively of people with terminal illness, bereavement difficulties and chronic diseases as well as depression or anxiety.

Next please . . .

A woman with multiple sclerosis realised that on a miracle day she would wake up in a bed on her own having had a good nights sleep and that she could then slide easily from her bed into a shower cubicle in her bedroom. She hadn't realised that her worry about her twitching legs keeping her husband awake had also spoilt her sleep, nor that she needed to get the occupational therapist round to look at further adjustments to her house.

Next please . . .

A woman whose daughter had died in a car accident the year before and whose son had taken an overdose as a result, hadn't realised that her life had become unhelpfully suspended. She needed to re-establish contact with her women friends and give herself the permission to laugh that her daughter would certainly have endorsed.

Next please . . .

A man with lung cancer was able to ask his wife for a small helping of smoked salmon for his lunch, knowing it would give her pleasure to give him a treat.

Both the choice of questions, as well as the language used to frame these, have considerable effects on the course of the consultation. The patient is led to reflect about the problem and the wider context. The clinician becomes increasingly curious about the feedback received which, in turn, inspires the inquiry. There are many different types of questions that can be asked to set in motion a process of reflection in the patient.

Some of the questions, particularly hypothetical ones, may seem odd, if not subversive. The clinician will have to wait for an appropriate moment to ask them. Many of the questions are comparative and use adverbs such as 'most' and 'least'. The choice of these words is deliberate in that it encourages the patient to look for

Practice task

- Ask your friend/partner about what to do next Sunday and the effects this may have on you and others, using reflexive questions.
- Choose five questions each from the seven categories of questions listed on pages 54–57.
- Interview one another and find out which questions affected you most.

and find differences in people's beliefs, actions and responses. In this way the patient may start questioning their own and various family members' belief systems and how these relate to the symptoms. Some questions are deliberately 'triadic', they are meant to encourage the patient to think about relationships between two people as observed through a third person. These questions also set up arbitrary scenarios (e.g. 'What would happen if X said this to Z?') with often utterly predictable results. 'Before' and 'after' questions can help to establish the connection a particular symptom may have in relation to a family event.

Next please . . .

Mrs S, aged 47, went to her health centre for yet another repeat prescription of sleeping tablets. The receptionist asked the practice nurse to have a conversation with her. It soon emerged that she had been quite low for a while. When pressed she said it was 'nothing to worry about'. The practice nurse did not give up but persisted and asked who was living in the home. It emerged that she and her husband were about to face an 'empty nest' as the result of their 18-year-old son going to university in another town. Mrs S tried to make light of this when she pointed out that this was 'normal and I really have no other worries'.

NURSE:	*'Does your husband know that you have sleeping problems?'*
MRS S:	*'I am not sure, he has his beers after dinner and then passes out.'*
NURSE:	*'Is that OK with you? Is that the way you want it?'*
MRS S:	*'Well . . . yes and no.'*
NURSE:	*'Was there a time when he didn't?'*
MRS S:	*'Yes, when we were younger . . . some years ago. We did have some fun.'*
Nurse:	*'Do you think he is worried about anything?'*
MRS S:	*'I wouldn't know.'*
NURSE:	*'If he was worried about something, what might it be?'*
MRS S:	*'He really loves our son. They have so much in common. He'll miss him.'*
NURSE:	*'More or less than you?'*
MRS S:	*'We both will, for different reasons.'*
NURSE:	*'Does he know that you think he is down because of that? Or does he know that you are also down about your son leaving, but for different reasons?'*
MRS S:	*'We don't talk a lot.'*
NURSE:	*'What would happen if you did?'*
MRS S:	*'We would probably both cry.'*
NURSE:	*'Would that be a good thing or a bad thing?'*

MRS S: 'It wouldn't be bad.'

NURSE: 'So, how could you start a conversation with him about that? What would be a
            good opening? What would be the best time you could broach the subject?'

MRS S: 'Well I could on Sunday morning. That's when there is a bit of time. But then there
            are the Sunday papers.'

NURSE: 'Who would be more tearful if you talked about missing your son – he or you?'

MRS S: 'I think he would be surprised about how I feel. I am quite depressed about it all.'

NURSE: 'If your son had been a fly on the wall, what might he think about the discussion
            we are having?'

MRS S: 'God alone knows. He'd be flattered to discover how important he is to us.'

NURSE: 'He doesn't know?'

MRS S: 'He never talks to me. He does to his dad, about football.'

NURSE: 'And what effect does that have on you?'

MRS R: 'Makes me feel worse.'

NURSE: [asks the next few questions, one by one, with Mrs S's responses omitted for space
            reasons]

            'How could you talk to him in such a way that he wouldn't make you feel worse?'

            'How would you have to start?'

            What would you expect his response to be?'

            'So if he says that, how could you reply in such a way that you don't give him a
            chance to be angry?'

            'Try this out, maybe this Sunday, and then come back next week and tell me how
            it went. How many sleepless nights is that going to give you?'

A whole range of different issues have been raised during this relatively brief conversation. The questions deliberately set out to explore connections between the presenting symptoms and family dynamics. They encourage the making of new links in the hope that this will make the patient see her predicament in a new light and allow her to mobilise some forces on the home front – as soon as the following Sunday.

Putting the problem in the chair – externalising questions

Usually we put our questions to our patients directly. But sometimes it is more effective to put the symptom or problem in the chair, as if it was separate from the person. This may at first sight seem a curious proposition, smacking of amateur dramatics. However, as mentioned in the last chapter, the technique of 'externalisation of problems' can be a useful way of personifying the problem a person experiences as oppressive. In this way the problem temporarily becomes a separate entity, external to the person. Often people can feel pretty bad about the fact that they do not seem to be able to beat off the illness. The illness and their sense of self seem to merge. Some of the language we use probably does not help. People who might have seen themselves as the bank manager, the welder, the father, the carer become simply a diabetic or a schizophrenic. Separating the symptom or the illness from the person can be perceived as both liberating and respectful and can lead to a sense of greater control over the illness or symptom.

Being afflicted by a chronic illness is usually a pervasive experience for the individual and the family. The sense of where the illness and the person begin and end gets blurred. The illness may get meanings ascribed to it that have no relation to its type or its severity, with resulting muddled thinking.

A number of writers (Griffith and Griffith 1992) use the metaphor of the illness being an elephant in the sitting room. It can feel so big that there is no room for anything else in the room. The elephant stops people seeing each other or watching TV, or even getting out of the room. It gets in the way of relationships. How to reduce the influence – or size – of the elephant can be a helpful metaphor. 'Putting the illness in the chair' is a technique to tackle these confusions.

Next please ...

Mrs F was the mother of a 13-year-old insulin-dependent diabetic boy called Brian. She had recently separated from Brian's father following an incident of severe physical violence between father and son. The diabetic liaison nurse was concerned that Brian's diabetes had spiralled hopelessly out of control, despite her persistent attempts at health education. Mrs F saw her GP for a consultation to reflect on what had happened and how things could be different in the future.

DR Y: 'I think we need to understand what's happened. I want us to do something that may seem a bit strange at first. Supposing we were to put Brian's diabetes in this chair over there, what would it look and feel like?'

MRS F   *[long pause, looks initially a bit puzzled]:* 'Like an enormous 6-foot syringe.'

DR Y: 'So when you look at that huge syringe, what does it make you feel like?'

MRS F: 'Really scared and completely useless. I am thinking: how can I help Brian put that in himself?'

DR Y: 'Has it always seemed that big?'

MRS F: 'Well no, not in the beginning. It's got out of proportion since his dad and I haven't been getting on. Actually the syringe reminds me of his dad – too much for me to cope with and painful.'

DR Y: 'So would I be right to think that in your mind there could be a muddle that when you are trying to help Brian with his diabetes, you're also thinking of his dad?'

MRS F: 'Yes. I suppose I'm cross with them both.'

DR Y: 'And if we put his dad in a separate chair to talk about your cross feelings about him, how big would the syringe look?'

MRS F   *[smiles]:* 'Absolutely normal size!'

DR Y: 'If Brian were here how big do you think he would say the syringe was?'

MRS F: 'I think normal size – it's really no big deal for him. It always amazes me how he just gets on with it.'

Following this (abbreviated) consultation the diabetic liaison nurse made contact with Brian and Mrs F. Diabetic control was re-established and has been maintained despite continuing difficulties over the separation.

Externalising illnesses, separating them for a few brief moments from their carriers, allows new perspectives to emerge.

Next please ...

Mr and Mrs B consulted their GP because Mrs B said Mr B was not taking responsibility for managing his multiple sclerosis and the impact that his urine incontinence had on her. She was furious that despite calmly talking to him and then ranting and railing, she had made no difference to his behaviour. He sat looking cheerfully passive in his wheelchair, while she was seething on the edge of her seat.

DR G: 'I'd be really interested to try a rather unusual conversation with you both to try to see this differently. Would that be OK?'

MR AND
MRS B: 'Yes.'

DR G: 'Supposing we put the whole of John's illness in that chair over there, quite separate from John as a person, what would that look like to each of you?'
            [pregnant pause]

MR B: 'Well it's just a little version of me and is something I know all the ins and outs of.'

MRS B: 'Well, that is amazing because for me it is a huge foggy cloud that is billowing out of the chair and is going to swallow me up.'

DR G: 'Is it hot, cold, smelly or anything else?'

MRS B: 'It's hot, steamy and . . . suffocating. It doesn't really smell.'

DR G: 'What have you been thinking, listening to your wife describe her experience of that MS over there?'

MR B: 'Well I'm amazed because it is so different an illness for her.'

DR G: 'What would have to happen for you to help her have the same view of your illness that you have?'

MR B: 'I really don't know . . . that is a puzzle. I suppose if I told her clearly what I wanted her to do for me that would help. Sometimes she guesses and gets it wrong and that's when she gets steamy. Really my illness is for me to look after.'

DR G: 'How do you think she could control the cloud for herself?'

MR B: 'Well I think that if she is relaxed and out and about enjoying herself my MS isn't as big a burden – she does forget to look after herself you know.'

MRS B: 'He's right really.'

DR G: 'The next time you both see the steamy cloud coming, what will you both do differently?'

MRS B: 'Go and take a break to cool off.'

MR B: 'I'd really be pleased if you did that without me having to say.'

DR G: 'John, supposing you got cross and steamy with the MS sitting there in that chair over there, all smug and self-satisfied, what would that be like? What would you say?'

MR B: 'I'd be really scared to in case it got out of control and overwhelmed me too.'

DR G: 'If it got out of control like your wife's steamy cloud, how long would it take to settle down?'

MR B: 'It would take a couple of days. I'd feel sad and sorry for myself – it is an unfair illness to have.'

DR G: 'Is it helpful to feel sad from time to time?'

MR B: 'It is really OK for me, but I hate it if it makes the steamy cloud come along for my wife, so I try and bottle it up.'

DR G: 'What have you been thinking, listening to John talk about his illness and his feelings?'

MRS B: 'Perhaps I should let him be when he is a bit down and not keep chivvying him because doing that makes my steamy cloud grow.'

Six weeks later the couple reported a considerable change in their relationship and in their relationship to the multiple sclerosis. Mr B confessed that he had been fighting off his need to accept his greater dependence on a wheelchair. He was actually getting out more than before. He prepared himself better for trips out and there had been no incontinent episodes. Mrs B spent more time out enjoying herself on her own and she reported that her 'steamy cloud' had now become manageable. They used the steamy cloud metaphor to enable their teenage son to talk about the MS and its effect on him. They had been worried that he would not be able to leave home, believing that his parents needed him with all the problems. A year later he left to go to college.

What is it that works with this approach? The relationships of the family members with a particular illness is temporarily changed as it assumes a life of its own. Once separate from its carrier, it becomes easier to express anger and other strong emotions to the illness, without feeling guilty about hurting the person. It operates on a symbolic and sometimes playful level that gives the family a different non-medical language to use to talk about and face the illness. Yet, there are so many, too many, questions and endlessly interesting answers. It is important not to think you can put more than one or two into a 10-minute consultation and also not to get too hung up on the idea that out there is the one magic right question that will solve everything. So, here are three questions for you! Are they going to 'solve' any of your problems?

Three questions for you

- Supposing you chose to put just one of the questions in this chapter to most of your patients in surgery tomorrow, which would you choose first?
- If you were to choose a category of questions to try the next day in one selected consultation, which would that be?
- Supposing you could talk further to a systemic practitioner about expanding your repertoire of questions, which further category would you choose to be tantalised by?

Practice task

Imagine a problem – or symptom – that you have or have had. Put it on another chair and have an imaginary conversation with it, questioning its very existence. Ask who feeds it and who allows it to have most influence on you.

The family within us – genograms

5

This chapter covers:
- Family patterns
- Family scripts
- Family narratives
- Constructing and using family trees
- Taking a new look at old stories

Family patterns and family scripts

We are all affected by our families of origin. They have not only passed on their genes, but also their beliefs, myths and implicit or explicit rules. Sometimes they have even passed on some of their illnesses and problems. When we team up with a partner we take on board his or her 'family luggage' and, if we have children, adopted or biological, we may well land them with it – and they can carry some of this through their life and pass it on to the next generation. Patterns of family relationships also tend to be transmitted from generation to generation. We cannot help but be influenced by what we have seen and experienced in our families of origin. Some of this is culturally mediated. Some of it is highly idiosyncratic within a given culture. With our children we may consciously wish to do the same – or the opposite – of what we were exposed to when being parented. But we may also be quite unaware of how we replicate familiar scripts – despite an intense conscious wish not to do so. And all of us, individuals and couples with or without children still take our own family patterns and beliefs and 'cultures' into every other nook and cranny of our lives: the way we react to the boss, how we treat friends and enemies, the way we think about washing our hands! In some way or other we take our families wherever we go.

Family beliefs, myths and scripts

Most families have their own myths, some of which may be referred to openly, others that are never identified as such, but are just woven into the tapestry of family life. Such myths tend to relate to many diverse issues, such as gender roles,

Myths – a definition

A series of fairly well-integrated beliefs shared by all the family members, concerning each other and their mutual positions in the family life. Beliefs that go unchallenged by everyone involved, in spite of the reality distortions that they may conspicuously imply (Ferreira 1963).

ideas about illness, family strengths and weaknesses. Myths inform the way we live, they co-write the scripts of family life. Our belief systems, our hopes and worries, our actions, our routines, how we relate to one another – all this is usually so predictable, as if scripted by invisible hands over generations. Family scripts are unwritten, of course. They are learned, usually over a period of many years, through repetition. Such scripts prescribe behaviours concerning the making and breaking of relationships, or how to bring up children, what roles the extended family has or what is generally permitted and what not.

Children mostly learn how to be parents from the direct experiences they had with their own parents, who in turn learned this from theirs. One generation later this can result either in *replicative* scripts, where a similar style of parenting is adopted, or in *corrective* scripts, where attempts are made to correct the alleged 'mistakes' of previous generations (Byng-Hall 1995). No matter whether they are replicative or corrective, family scripts can be like strait-jackets, even if there is no conscious awareness of their presence or their restrictive effects. And here is the interesting thing: physical or psychological symptoms are frequently the only signs that people have become fixed in their scripted roles. Illness is one way to break away from repressive patterns – but at a cost.

- 'So who taught you to worry about things the way you do?'
- 'Now where did you learn that, to always be apologising for yourself?'
- 'Did you get that idea about eating from your mother or your father?'

Looking at family scripts and examining these helps people to become aware of trans-generational patterns of health and illness (Bowen 1978). Constructing diagrams of the generations of a family – so-called family trees, or genograms – helps us to become aware of such patterns and permits the identification of possible ways of getting away from being 'typecast' and stuck in uncomfortable roles. By having a closer look at the various people in the family drama, it becomes possible to examine and challenge some of the fantasies or beliefs that cause current problems. It also allows histories from the past to be rewritten, with new resolutions and endings.

The genogram is an excellent tool for eliciting stories about families or, as it is now more fashionably worded, for creating 'family narratives'. It helps to establish the patient's life – and illness – story. From it new explorations are possible. History does not have to repeat itself – even though Mrs D is at a point at which she could buy into an old script.

Next please . . .

Mrs D, mother of 4-year-old Natalie, asked for a meeting with the health visitor whom she had last met when Natalie was in her infancy. She said that her daughter gave her a lot of worries and that she was now very worried about not being a good mother. The examples Mrs D gave about Natalie's behaviour did not seem particularly concerning to the health visitor. Not knowing much about the family, she felt a bit at a loss and asked Mrs D, 'Is it OK if I ask a bit about your family background?' Mrs D told her about her husband and her unmarried sister. The health visitor asked whether it would be all right for her to do a 'family tree . . . so that I can understand who's around in your life, who is important or has been important'. When talking about her parents and grandparents, Mrs D revealed that her grandmother had died when giving birth to Mrs D's mother. She said that her mother had always felt 'odd' and that she had very little self-confidence. She suffered from recurrent depression and had to be hospitalised on many occasions. With some further questioning she remembered the first time her mother had been admitted: 'I was about as old as my daughter is now'. The health visitor hardly needed to prompt Mrs D to make the connection, as Mrs D asked: 'Do you think this has anything to do with my daughter's behaviour?'

Family narratives

The field of narrative therapy (White and Epston 1990, White 1997, Morgan 2000) has made significant contributions that are applicable to primary care settings. It is based on the idea that everybody tries to give meaning to their experiences. Our daily lives are full of little and bigger events, which we weave together over time and which eventually form a story. Narrative therapists say that events are linked in sequence, across time and according to a plot. It could be said that we understand and live our life through stories. There are, of course, many simultaneous – and at times conflicting – stories we have about our lives and relationships. These may include stories about what we are good at and what not; stories about our achievements and failures; about our ambitions and abilities; about our interests and dislikes. How we link these stories together – and which ones we believe to be more true than others – depends very much on how we have linked events together and what meaning has been attributed to them.

> CLINICIAN: 'Which stories about yourself are more helpful to believe right now? If you completely believed your grandparents' stories about yourself what would that mean for you?'

The genogram is a powerful tool for exploring illness and relationship stories, and how past patterns come to influence the presence.

Medical myths

There is a whole category of myths that relate specifically to beliefs about illness and health and within that a category of medical myths to which clinicians have wittingly or unwittingly contributed. Hardwick (1989) has written a very helpful account of medical myths. He characterises a number of different distortions (we might now say alternative ideas) that occur:

* About the presence of a condition
* About the severity of a condition
* About the recovery or lack of recovery from a condition
* About the way a condition manifests itself
* About the causation of a condition
* About the treatment of a condition
* About the transmission of a condition.

Here are just a few to whet your appetite:

* 'If we did not cook special foods for him, he would starve to death.'
* 'If we don't give in, he will have a "fit" and might die.'
* 'You should always wrap up a temperature/sweat out a cold.'

Here is another familiar one:

* 'If you hadn't sent me in when you did the doctors say, I would have died.' Or the more familiar, 'The doctors at the hospital said I was right to ignore your advice – I was hours away from death.'

Hardwick also gives many examples of iatrogenic (and this includes nurses as well as doctors!) myths:

The parents of Stuart, a highly anxious teenager, overheard their GP say 'psychotic' while dictating a referral letter. The prescription of medication further confirmed the family's fears that Stuart was taking after a mentally ill relative. The family became more frightened of Stuart and mounted a 24-hour vigil over him. Not surprisingly, Stuart's symptoms increased, confirming the need for the vigil.

And the seed

Try identifying one medical myth in tomorrow's consultations and one in your family of origin.

Next please . . .

Mr B consulted his GP because of some diffuse anxiety-related symptoms. When asked about his family of origin, he said he was a 'typical middle child'. His older brother had always been seen by everyone as the 'brain' of the family, achieving well in school and at university. His younger brother was nicknamed 'Mr Charming', making everyone laugh from early on. He pursued a successful career in the theatre. Mr B described himself as a 'shy', 'retiring' and a 'peacemaking' person. When asked whether he also had acquired a childhood nickname, Mr B revealed, with some embarrassment, that he used to be called 'Softie'. Asked to elaborate his story of being a 'softie', Mr B spoke about how he was 'right in the middle between my two strong brothers', being 'a soft target' for their jokes. He also remembered that he had been told that he was 'soft in the brain' and somehow this had stuck in his head. When asked, by referring to the different persons on a diagram of the family – the genogram – who in the family had shared the view of the brothers, Mr B pointed accusingly at both his parents, the paternal grandparents, various uncles and aunts. The GP then asked about the maternal grandparents and Mr B's voice almost broke when he said: 'They were different. They always told me I was strong . . . I was special.'

The dominant story about Mr B in his early life was that of someone who was soft, a walkover. Over time more and more events and experiences were selected into the dominant plot, with this then becoming seeming 'reality'. Mr B eventually believed the stories about him. It is difficult to get away from such typecasting and plots. Yet, our lives consist of more than just one story – different stories can be told about the same event. If Mr B was asked to give examples of events that did not fit the story of a soft and feeble person, he might have initial difficulties. However, if he was asked what his maternal grandparents had to say about him, he might tap into an alternative narrative.

Putting the family tree together

Some practices and health centres now ask newly registered patients to fill in a form which contains a family tree. This is useful in that it helps the clinician to see at one glance who is in the family, and it can be a good and efficient way of joining with the patient(s). But be careful that it does not become a routine 'fact'-gathering tool, because it is the very process of constructing the genogram together with the patient that is a creative exchange. The genogram:

- Combines biomedical and psychosocial information
- Is an excellent database for future reference
- Emphasises the clinician's interest in the context of their patient's life
- Produces unexpected stories
- Makes connections between seemingly unconnected events and persons
- Reveals trans-generational patterns of disease and problem behaviours
- Places the presenting problem in an historical context
- Arouses new curiosity in the clinician about the patient, and for the patient in themselves
- Has diagnostic and therapeutic value as well as building a better relationship between clinician and patient.

To construct a genogram, a good-sized piece of paper is needed. It is the clinician who draws the family tree, with the help of the patient. The developing map becomes the centre of interest, with both focusing on it. Here are some opening comments the clinician can make:

> *I don't really seem to know much about you, could you tell me a bit about yourself and your family? I will draw this up together with you, like a family tree, so that I can remember who is who and how everyone fits in.*

> *We don't seem to have been able to help your pains so far; perhaps it might help if we looked together at the patterns of illness in your family?*

> *We seem to keep investigating the headaches and not come up with an explanation. I wonder whether it would be helpful to go back and see what illnesses have been in your family and see if there are any clues in that?*

> *I realise I know a lot about you but at present it doesn't seem to make much sense to either of us. I would like to pretend that I know nothing about you and start afresh. Let's draw a family tree.*

Watch the non-verbals

During the process of creating the family tree with patients, it is important to be aware of their verbal and non-verbal feedback. Painful issues can be tackled, provided the clinician is sensitive:

- 'You look a bit tense when you talk about him.'
- 'That must have been very difficult.'
- 'How awful, having to cope with that amount of illness.'
- 'You were only 10 when your mother died. Do you remember anything about that time?'
- 'You mean you were born after two miscarriages? I wonder what that meant to your parents.'
- 'You have the same name as your uncle. Are there any similarities?'
- 'I notice that you were born shortly after your mother's father died. Was that significant? Or, what effect do you think this may have had on how you were seen?'

Such comments, which underline or emphasise certain events, are possible openings for a new – or old and buried – story to emerge. However, it is up to the patient to decide whether they want to talk about some of these issues in more detail. The questions are probes to help patients to draw attention to certain issues, inviting them to reflect on these anew.

Most clinicians will have had some experience with drawing a family tree. There are many different ways of doing this and personal styles and annotations vary a great deal. A family tree can consist of three or four generations joined together, with detailed information on each member as well as important relationships between

them. In practice this is often not possible in one consultation. At times it is sufficient to look just at two generations, to get to know the family and some of the issues.
    In order to create a family tree, symbols are used:

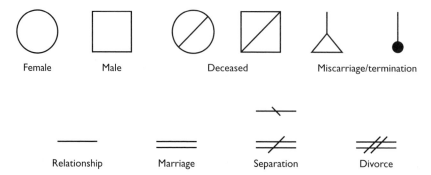

Figure 5.1(i)

The clinician can start by saying: 'This is you, Mrs K, and I shall draw you as a
circle, here in the middle of the paper.' Her first name, date of birth, and any other
information can be noted down, next to the circle denoting Mrs K. 'Tell me about
your partner.' If Mrs K has a partner then a horizontal line is drawn and a square
placed at the other end of that line.

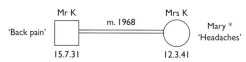

Figure 5.1(ii)

The next question could be: 'Do you have children?' They are placed below the
marriage line. Miscarriages, terminations or stillbirths can also be entered if appropriate.

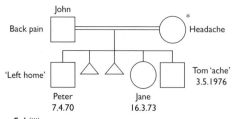

Figure 5.1(iii)

Previous marriages or other important relationships, children from other partners,
can also be entered ('Are there or were there any other important relationships that

you might want to mention . . . or children from previous relationships?'). It can be helpful to insert dates of all marriages, separations and deaths.

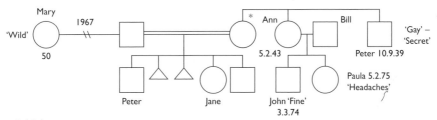

Figure 5.1(iv)

The next step is to move to the third generation: 'And what about your parents?'

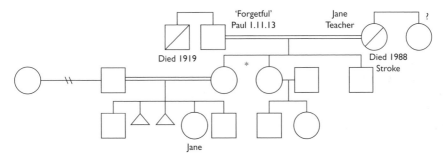

Figure 5.1(v)

Getting all these details can take time but if you do get around to doing it then you will find it is occasionally very useful. Dates often connect people with past events: 'So you were actually born the same week that your mother's father died. I wonder what impact that has had on you or your mother?'

To enter the area of health, the clinician can ask whether each person is 'fit and well?' If there are any known illnesses and specific problems, they can be written next to the person. The clinician may then wish to proceed and ask about the third generation – 'And what about your parents?' Once this is completed, the tree of the partner's family of origin can be filled in, if appropriate.

Clinicians vary a great deal in how they construct these family trees. Some note down next to each family member specific information regarding illnesses, birth weights, occupations, nicknames, geographical data, socio-economic status, significant relationships, religion, ethnicity and cultural issues (Hardy and Laszloffy 1995). Whilst one could spend hours doing this, in practice there is usually not that much time. This forces clinicians to make some decisions as to what to go for, remembering that this technique is above all meant to benefit the patient, rather than becoming a research project in its own right.

Genograms

Here are a few tips on how to do genograms:

*   Plan how much time you can afford – it is possible to construct a genogram in 10 minutes.
*   Remember, patients usually come back. There is no need to hurry. You can always continue next time.
*   Lots of families are quite complicated, with multiple partners and lots of siblings. It can be worth asking a few general questions about the family so that you don't run out of space on the page!
*   Start with medical information; in a primary care context, patients usually find this least threatening.
*   Explore around one theme, preferably one that has aroused some emotion in the patient.
*   Encourage the patient to talk about the relationships between the people represented on the genogram.
*   Try to make it a joint exploration. This takes the pressure off you to 'solve' the puzzle and encourages the patient to be more active.

Making the connections

Once the skeleton of the family tree has been erected, a series of comments or questions can be put to link the presenting problem or symptom with family issues. Such connections must not be forced by making apparently 'clever' statements, but can be explored in more tentative ways.

Examples of questions are:

*   'Show me who else in the family has had pains like you?'
*   'Who can you talk about your pains to?'
*   'What happens when you do? Who of these people here on your family tree are most/least sympathetic?'
*   'Who of these do you try to keep the problem secret from?'
*   'Why? What would happen if they found out?'
*   'Who of these never talk about their problems? Who goes on about their illnesses?'
*   'Tell me about that relationship [pointing to it on the tree]: how does he get on with her?'
*   'Most families have someone with a drinking problem. Who is it in yours?'
*   'Who is the scapegoat/drop-out in your family?'
*   'Who of these people taught you to be shy/anxious/angry/depressive?'
*   'What sort of things do people die from on your side?'
*   'You don't seem to know much about that bit of the family – why is that?'
*   'You all seem very close/distant. Is that how you see it? What is that like for you?'

- 'Have you noticed that these two things happened at the same time?' [e.g. your mother divorced your father the same time your son was born]
- 'Had it struck you before that the oldest child always leaves home at a very early age?'
- 'Is there anyone or anything else that should be on that family tree? Or anyone else we should know about?'
- 'Is there any incest on this family tree?'
- 'If you could change one thing in your family, what would you change?'

These and other questions tend to stimulate a process of self-reflection in patients: 'How is it that we behave in this way? What makes us think that things inevitably happen in a particular way? What would happen if we tried things differently?'

In the process of co-constructing a genogram with the clinician, many patients make new discoveries. It is the weaving of new connections, via reflecting on questions, which can help the patient to put the pieces of the jigsaw puzzle together. At times some pieces are missing which then requires the patient to do some 'homework': 'Who would you have to talk to so that you can fill in this blank space . . . maybe your aunt? Well, how could you get her to talk about this?' or 'Why don't you find out from your husband what happened?' If the patient takes some of these questions or even the half-completed genogram home, then there is a good chance that other family members will get involved in the exploration. In fact, it is quite possible that next time round the spouse will demand to come to the surgery so that he can 'correct' the family tree. In this way the genogram has become a kind of catalyst, making it possible for old beliefs to be questioned and new ways of looking at old predicaments to take place.

However, constructing genograms is not always a simple and straightforward affair. Some patients can get upset as old wounds are opened up. Questions need to be alternated with empathic statements, watching the patient very carefully for any signs of discomfort and acknowledging these: 'It looks as if you find it very difficult to talk about this now. Maybe you want to stop, maybe you want to take a break.' This slows down and focuses the conversations, allowing for new or old stories to be told. It is also important and caring – letting the patient know that their distress is being noticed.

Some more practical considerations – it's not all magic

Genograms can be immensely powerful tools for exploring families, beliefs, myths and patterns. They can be 'magic'. But they can also just be handy aids to slightly better consulting. Having a genogram in the notes and being able to scan it before the patient walks in can refresh parts of the brain another examination of the notes will not reach! 'Oh yes, now I remember about the previous partner he had.' 'I had completely forgotten about that miscarriage she had two years before she married him, I wonder. . . .' 'Look at all the people with heart disease in this family – what sort of impact must that be having?'

Just starting the process of drawing a genogram with a patient involves you in a collaborative act, which can of itself help change the dynamic of the consultation. Nothing much may appear to be revealed by the partial tree that you have drawn but messages have been transmitted about how current symptoms and family events may be connected. You may find yourself drawing a tree with someone only to discover that you know other members of their family, and had no idea they were connected. New ideas about what may be going on pop up.

Next please . . .

Mrs P came to see her GP with low mood after the breakup of her marriage. A brief family tree revealed she was the younger of two children to Mr and Mrs E. Her mother had had a depressive illness for many years and was looked after by an organically minded psychiatrist. Both her maternal grandparents were dead. Her paternal grandparents were still alive and the grandfather had bad heart disease. Mrs P revealed that she had been abused by a maternal uncle. She herself had had post-natal depression. The GP was not sure if doing the family tree helped much but Mrs P got over her divorce and seemed to be doing well.

Some years later the GP, while seeing Mrs P for a routine pill check, reviewed her family tree only to discover that he now knew both her parents and paternal grandparents well now. The father struggled with stress and anger about work colleagues and his body was a mass of tightness and atypical chest pains. The GP was seeing him all too regularly. The grandfather was struggling with severe heart disease and multiple other problems and had had several close calls with death. The GP immediately began to generate tentative hypotheses about depression, anger, back and chest pain, and sexual abuse. He wasn't sure what to do with the hypotheses but maybe next time he saw the father he might steer the inevitable conversation about the work colleagues around to thinking about how anger was managed in his life?

Where to put them and how to record?

Record keeping in primary care is varied but increasingly computerised. This presents both challenges and possibilities. Genograms can be stored on the inside cover of A4 notes, so they appear as soon as the file is opened. You can scan them into electronic records and search for them with a marker. There are software programs for constructing family trees, but to our knowledge these are insufficiently flexible and user friendly to be used in real time in primary care consultations, although we are always interested to hear if someone has managed this yet. The ideal would be the ability to bring up the family tree at the click of a switch in just the same way as past medical history is revealed. You may be inclined to give them to the person with whom you have been talking, although it is often useful to keep a copy for your records. Some clinicians simply keep a file of all the ones they have done and refer to them whenever they need. It is worth having a discussion with other clinicians in the team and seeing whether you can adopt a practice policy on the regular use of genograms in the notes.

When is it appropriate to try one?

It will not surprise you to learn that 'any time' is the preferred answer! But in particular, any time when you feel that you or the patient might be stuck, every time you feel like widening the lens, is a time to consider doing a family tree.

The genogram with the whole family

A more advanced way of using family trees as exploratory tools is to involve the whole family. They can all, on a big piece of paper or on a board, draw their family. The clinician may ask the parents whether they would want the children to start drawing whatever they know about the family. It is often startling to see how much small children know and this can be quite a surprise to the parents who may have always believed that they had shielded their offspring from some important, allegedly 'harmful' secrets. Starting with the children also allows the clinician to form a picture of family interactions, for example, how the children obtain information from their parents, how much the children are controlled or interrupted by the parents, who is the main parental caretaker, or in what way father and mother give different signals to their children. By giving the children the lead, it is possible to find out how much they know themselves and it is then left to the parents whether and how to fill in the missing gaps. However, it is very important to state at the outset that the parents are in charge of their children and that it is up to them to stop any topics or questions which they regard as inappropriate or harmful. This deals with an important issue, namely that patients often feel that clinicians are entitled to every possible piece of knowledge about the family – including intimate details about their sex lives. It is good practice for clinicians to repeatedly state in consultations: 'I may want to ask you quite a few questions. I hope these questions are sensitive, but if I ask an inappropriate question, or a question you don't want to answer, feel free to do so – or just say "pass".'

When children are present, clinicians must be sensitive not to pressurise parents into talking about issues they do not want to discuss in front of their offspring. Clinicians must also be prepared to create a boundary when families persist in talking inappropriately in front of the children. Giving parents the responsibility for deciding what can and what cannot be discussed confirms them in their parental authority. Sensitive clinicians will at various points of a consultation remind the patient or family: 'Is it all right if I ask that question?' or 'Please feel free to let me know if I ask questions that are uncomfortable or if I get you to talk about things you'd rather not talk about' or 'I leave it entirely up to you to decide whether you want to talk about this in front of your children or not'.

Next please . . .

Janice consulted her family doctor. She was 35 and had discovered she was pregnant for the first time and she was in a great quandary. She had never used contraception in the 10 years of her relationship with Bill. A double appointment was set aside to look at doing a family tree to help understand all the strands of influences involved in making the decision to terminate the pregnancy or not.

This is what the consultation revealed: Janice was the fifth child out of six. She had a sister 15 years younger than her, who had just had a baby. All her other siblings had had children. She had felt quite apart from them all as when she was 15 she had felt a profound disgust and embarrassment at her mother having a baby, and had left home to live with her maternal grandmother. Now she wanted to feel part of her family again. Bill was the younger brother in a very dispersed unemotional family where there had been much unhappiness. His brother had a drink problem and his father had died of alcoholic liver disease. His parents had separated when he was 16. He wasn't sure if his mother was alive. Janice felt that Bill would struggle to be a father because he had had no good experiences to go on. She worried about the future of their relationship if she had the baby because he couldn't talk to her about the pregnancy. The more she tried the more he clammed up.

Here are some of the questions the GP asked:

*   'Supposing you stopped pursuing Bill as a potential father and let him adjust slowly and in his own time and way to the notion of parenthood, how long would it take for him to want to talk to you?'
*   'Supposing you understood that you could be a good and confident mother because of your close family and good experiences, what would you decide?'
*   'What do you think would be the effect on Bill of seeing you being a good mother? Who else is there in your family to help Bill think about how to be a father?'
*   'In five years' time what would the pattern of family relationships look like if you kept/didn't keep the baby?'

Family trees are marvellous visual aids. Furthermore, they are like 'transitional objects', out there between the clinician and patient. Both pore over it, examining patterns and histories. During the process of being asked circular questions, the patient is temporarily assuming a meta-position, looking at their own family life from a different vantage point, while the clinician is curious about the stories seemingly jumping out of the picture. Both clinician and patient co-evolve new perspectives and therefore the beginnings of new stories. This is very therapeutic for most patients.

Next please …

Mr M presented with atypical chest pains exactly three years after his father had died of a myocardial infarction. Physical examination was normal, as was an exercise ECG. His choles-terol was slightly raised. The practice nurse decided to complete a genogram looking for other risk factors to help with assessing the need for primary prevention of cardiovascular disease. She was very struck by the story of bereavement/loss that emerged. Mr M's eldest son was leaving home to go away to university, leaving two younger sisters and a much younger brother at home. Mr M was really upset at his departure as he had a close relationship with this boy. The practice nurse wondered whether there had been any other losses in the family. Mr M told her about his cousin (his only cousin) who had died in a road accident at the same age as his son was. He also talked about how his father's mother had died when his father was 4 and how his father had been brought up by a fierce spinster aunt. He and his little brother had clung together as their father hadn't been able to cope or protect them from the aunt's tongue. Mr M thought his father had never really got on properly with his mother as he was scared of women and that he had transmitted this fear of women to him. Mr M admitted he didn't really get on with his wife and was worried with his son leaving home about what it would be like at home with her. Mr M's chest pains settled at this time, though over the next few years he developed angina. He separated from his wife and entered a gay relationship. He often referred to the genogram as having helped him understand in one go how his muddled feelings developed. The practice nurse wondered about the powerful story of male relation-ships born out of loss and whether that could make someone gay.

To summarise, the *process* of constructing the genogram is in many ways more important than the result – even though it is rewarding to have a comprehensive family tree at the end, to be filed in the case notes. Historical information is above all useful in consultations when it comes alive through the interaction of patient, clinician and the family.

Genogram summary

1 Do your own genogram and your partner's or your friend's. To describe your family you could write 10 lines beginning 'In my house ...'.

2 Imagine the sorts of questions that a doctor might ask you in a consultation. Identify which areas you would rather not be probed about.

3 Ask five consecutive patients about the health of their parents, compare it with what is already recorded and note the effect of taking this history on the rest of the consultation.

4 Invite first-time mothers-to-be to complete a genogram (their own and their partner's). Try predicting what the closeness and distance patterns will be for this new family.

This chapter covers:
- How to construct family circles
- How to make sense of them
- How to use them as tools for change

Sometimes it can be very helpful to view life from a different vantage point, as from close-up one often cannot see the wood for the trees. For example, being able to see the Earth from space has enabled us to see our 'home' in the round, as it were. Moreover, it has helped scientists to investigate and understand patterns of life on our planet. When it comes to personal relationships, we can equally benefit from taking a look at ourselves from outside. There are various ways in which we can construct maps of our life and interactions. We have seen how useful a family tree can be as a map of the territory. The Family Circles Method (Geddes and Medway 1977) and other related techniques (Bing 1970, Burns and Kaufman 1970) are another set of excellent tools to help patients examine their own lives and relationships in new ways.

The Family Circles Method is a quick and graphic way of gathering, assessing and working with personal and family information, as seen by one or more members of a family. It is particularly useful with individual patients, but can also be used with a couple or a family. It helps clinicians to get another perspective of a patient's life situation and predicaments. Such maps not only allow us to pinpoint where people are, but also where they have come from and where they might go in the future. The purpose of using mapping exercises such as the Family Circles Method is to help patients to connect current problems or illness with persons from the present and the past, as well as with other contextual issues, such as passions, interests, culture and religion. This not only adds a new dimension to the understanding of a patient's living contexts and the various dilemmas, but also provides a concrete starting point for making changes in their personal life and relationships. The technique also recognises that some people prefer to approach problem solving in a visual way. Not everyone is good at just talking about relationships – seeing them drawn is a very powerful and compelling tool.

The Family Circles Method asks individuals to draw or construct a schematic diagram of their life – composed of family, friends, interests and passions. It maps, in spatial relationships, people and interests not revealed in genograms. It provides a graphic and visual account of current life pressures, permitting patient and clinician to highlight specific problem areas, to identify strategies for change and to consider the implications of change. In this way the patient and the presenting problem(s) are being placed in context, thus opening another way of viewing relationships and how they help or hinder symptoms and illnesses. In practice the patient is asked to draw circles and circles within circles.

Drawing circles

A patient can create a family circle drawing in as little as three minutes. Once the method has been explained, the clinician leaves the patient to get on with the task of representing their life on paper. Depending on the circumstances, there are a number of ways in which clinicians can introduce the Family Circles Method:

- 'Somehow I don't seem to be able to get to the core of your problem, so perhaps it might help if we tried a new tack.'
- 'I don't know how to help you at the moment, so I would like to suggest we tried a new approach and looked at things from a different perspective.'
- 'Your problem seems to involve several people. Maybe we should try and understand how they are all connected with you.'
- 'Before we label this as a psychological problem (or call it 'gastritis' or ME), it might be worth exploring the possibility that this is to do with relationships.'
- 'Maybe we should explore whether anything in your life at the moment contributes to it.'

The clinician then draws a large circle on a piece of paper and instructs the patient as follows:

> *I am interested in you, your family and what is important to you. Let's imagine that this circle stands for your life as it is now. I would like you to draw in some smaller circles to represent all the other people important to you – family members, friends, enemies, neighbours, whoever you like. People can be inside or outside this large circle, they can be touching, overlapping or far apart. They can be large or small depending on how important they are to you. Anyone you think should be on this piece of paper, alive or not, family or not – just put them in. Do remember to put yourself in as well.*
>
> *Also put in other important areas of your life, such as work, hobbies, your God, or dog, or whatever. Put an initial on each circle so that you can iden-tify it later. And also, and that's important, put the illness – or your symptoms – in the circle – wherever you think they belong. And don't worry how you do it – there are no right or wrong circles, just do it the way you think it's best. Why don't you now take three minutes to do it, just by yourself and we can both have a look at it afterwards?*

The patient is then asked to complete the circles alone. Whilst the patient is engaged in this task, the clinician should not observe, but should carry out some other minor activity, such as doing some administration, give in to the tyranny of preventative health care and review what, if anything, else 'needs' to be done for this patient at another time, or sign some prescriptions, etc. This signals to the patient that it is their job to complete the task. It is useful to give a time limit that is on the short side (no more than 3–5 minutes). This results in the patient being more spontaneous rather than carefully editing what they might or might not put on paper.

Working with the circles

The first thing to remember is that this is not a projective test, with the clinician making clever interpretations on what he or she believes the picture reveals. Instead, this method needs to be seen as an entry ticket, a way designed to get the patient to think and talk about their own life.

To this effect the patient is first asked to explain the picture ('Would you like to tell me who is who and what is what?'). Some patients find this easier than others. They may just name the various circles and people and say little else. There is no need to intervene at this stage. If the patient is very hesitant, it may be necessary to encourage elaboration ('And who or what is this circle?'). Generally patients are not reluctant to talk about themselves and their lives, but they may need a bit of guidance and probing initially. The clinician, however, has to remain in a listening position, encouraging the patient to tell their story about the circles. Patients sometimes hesitate initially, they may look sad or happy when talking about one particular circle, they sometimes almost talk too much. All the clinician does at this stage is to listen with interest, making mental notes of what sounds like important information. This allows space for some questions that can be asked at a later stage.

Continuing to explore

Once the patient has given their account, the clinician can then follow up: 'Do you mind if I ask you some questions about this circle?' This is an opening for asking questions about specific aspects of the drawing. For example, it is possible to enquire as to whether there was any significance in the fact that some circles were bigger than others – or that quite a few are overlapping. These tentative, enquiring questions can trigger thoughts, without implying that the clinician 'knows' something the patient is not aware of. It is rather reminiscent of that phrase 'I don't know what I know until I hear myself say it'. Or in this case 'I don't know what I think until I see myself draw it'. The responses provide a picture of some aspects of the patient's life, the people in it and the various interests – or lack thereof. The clinician can then enquire about the space between people, the relative closeness and distance of certain relationships, about how work and other areas of life might affect various relationships.

A way of proceeding from here is to ask an open question: 'How do you like this picture? Are you happy with it?' This invites the patient to reflect on the overall picture as well as commenting on specifics. Many patients say that they found doing this exercise very helpful, thinking that they had a very rich and full life. Others express their surprise about how crowded or how empty their lives seem to be. Instead of just tuning into the details of the circles, they may make some more general statements about themselves, their lives and those involved in them. This can be a therapeutic shift of perspective.

There are patients who immediately want to change what they have drawn. They will say that things were 'wrong' or 'not true'. This may be evidence of a process of thinking having been triggered. It can also be a sign of a tendency to perfectionism, or a stance of never being happy with what one has done. The clinician can pick this up: 'I notice you are not quite satisfied with what you have done. Is this an exception or do you find yourself often wishing to change things?' Depending on the feedback from the patient, the clinician may follow this up by enquiring how easy or difficult it is for the patient to change things in their life.

There are various other ways of encouraging reflection: 'Looking at this picture now, is there anything that strikes you as being surprising?' 'I notice that this circle is very close to that one – can you tell me about that?' 'There seems to be a lot of space between circle A and C – is this just a coincidence or would you care to tell me about that?' Patients may well reply that a particular circle 'wasn't meant to be so big' or 'so small' and ask the clinician not to read anything too much into the drawing. Clinicians need to accept what patients say and not challenge it. It is not an aim of the Family Circles Method to convince patients of some hitherto unknown relationship conflicts or specific family dynamics, but to enable them to make such connections themselves, finding out for themselves rather than it being interpreted by an 'expert'.

Once a patient has started talking about the various circles and how and why there are certain spaces or overlaps between them, why one is bigger than another, why some are close and others may be even outside the main big circle, then it might be useful to reiterate the question: 'So, when you look at this picture, are you happy with it? Is there anything you might want to change – not just in the picture but also perhaps in real life? How would you like it to be different? How could you make that happen?'

Exploring relationships

In this way the drawing is used as a metaphor – the patient is encouraged to think more generally about relationship issues and whether and how changes might be brought about. Some patients provide spontaneous answers. Others fall silent and look puzzled and the clinician can then use circular questions to get the patient to reflect on change and its implications.

> *May I ask you a question: What would happen if you got closer to your mother? What if you told your wife that she should talk less to her own mother? How would that change this picture?*

> *I notice that you have put two circles outside the big circle. Can you tell me about that? Was there a time when you would have put these circles inside the big one? What happened? Might there be a time when these circles might get back inside? What would need to be different?*

As both patient and clinician look at the drawing, the clinician can point at various circles and trace the connections between various persons: 'So, if this relationship changed – what would happen to that one? If your wife's relationship with her mother was less close – what would that do to your wife's relationship with you? What might she want from you?'

If both clinician and patient examine the drawing together, they both look at the patient's life from another perspective. It is likely that, from this bird's eye perspective, the patient will see things not noticed before. For example, it may be revealed that if one relationship changes, another may need to do the same.

Exploring the illness

If things become too uncomfortable or intense for the patient, the clinician may turn to examine the symptom or illness and its impact on the family. If the patient has not drawn the place of the illness, the clinician may say:

> *I know you have been plagued by your illness for a very long time. If you had to put the illness (symptom) into this picture – where might you place it? Whom does the illness affect most? What relationships does it get in the way of? If it got bigger or worse, which relationships might be affected next?*

Focusing the patient on the picture and allocating a 'site' for the illness can often make its power and influence very clear. Questions alluding to change will get the patient to think further about the illness and its effects.

> *Let us imagine that by some piece of magic we are able to shrink the illness, to make it much smaller, much less powerful. Which things or persons in your life would get bigger? Which relationships might get closer – or more distant?*

The 'externalisation' of the symptom, problem or illness (see also Chapters 3 and 4) is a technique that makes these come alive as active players in people's lives. In this way the illness becomes a 'partner', affecting not only the sufferer but also other people. The illness has a life of its own. Apart from getting patients to consider the effects of illness on various relationships, it is also helpful to focus on other areas of life: 'If there was less of illness, what would you do more of (pointing at various hobbies or activities on the drawing)? Would you garden more? See friends? Spend more time in the office? Give up the church?'

Exploring time

Time is a major context that affects people's lives. The Family Circles Method permits exploration of change over time. Looking at a particular drawing and raising the question as to how this may have looked differently before illness struck can make meaningful connections. 'Before' and 'after' questions (described in Chapter 4) allow past and hypothetical future scenarios to be explored.

> *If we had met two years ago, before you ever had these symptoms, and I had asked you to do this drawing – how might you have drawn it then? You can show me on this drawing what might have been different – or you can do an entirely new picture.*

Many patients find this a fascinating task. It need not be illness focused – it could look at specific relationships before and after another significant event, perhaps the arrival of a new baby, the breakdown of a marriage, or the death of an elderly family member. Looking at your life through this lens opens up new perspectives. Something very similar can be done about the future:

What would you like this picture to look like in a year's time? How would you rearrange the circles to make these changes? If there was one thing you would want to be different, one little change you could make here on this piece of paper, what would it be? What's the first thing you need to do to move on? So, when and how are you going to go about it?

Most patients enjoy playing around with making certain circles bigger and realising that at the same time some other circles might have to get smaller, so that their life – or at least the picture of it – does not get too overcrowded.

- 'I notice that if you make these changes, there is going to be quite a lot of space on your picture here. What's going to occupy this space?'
- 'This circle, your child – you have drawn it so that it is between you and your husband. Does that cause problems or is it the way you want it?'
- 'There is a big hole in your life there. What does that mean? Do you feel you want to do something about that?'
- 'I see that work takes up most of your life. Is that the way you want it? If there was less work, which of these circles would become bigger?'
- 'It looks as though your children are at an age when, soon, they will all have left home. What difference will that make to the picture?'
- 'I note your mother is important, and she is getting older and is ill. How will the circles change when she dies?'
- 'What would have to change on this picture to make it possible for some of your hopes for the future to come true? Show me just where you might want to start?'

The Family Circles Method can be used to identify and set specific goals. It enables patients to look at themselves in new ways. It is not the clinician who identifies dysfunction or problems, but it is through the reflective way in which the interview is conducted that the patient becomes more aware of the potential for change in their own life and the family system. Patients are encouraged to make sense of the drawings themselves. If anyone is to 'interpret' what they mean it is the patient and *not* the clinician. Most patients will leave such a consultation feeling that something, maybe even everything, has become connected.

So far we have explained the usefulness of this method by employing the medium of a drawing. Another way of doing something fairly similar is to ask the patient to place objects (for example, different size shells, pebbles, buttons) on a piece of paper on which the clinician has drawn a big circle. The advantages of objects, such as buttons, is not only that they have different sizes and colours, but that they can be moved about on the paper. This is very dynamic, with the clinician being able to demonstrate that when one piece moves, others often have to follow by necessity.

Supposing I asked you to replace this big brown button, which you have told me stands for your work, with this small bright button, how does life look like for you? And what might take its place? How does the picture change if I moved this button (which you told me is your sister who is so demanding) right out of the centre and to one side? Show me what your life would look like. Just move the relevant buttons.

The Family Circles Method can fit neatly into a 10- or 20-minute consultation. It is, however, unlikely that all the issues raised can be discussed within that time scale. In fact, it is often not even desirable to do so. The patient can continue with the exploration on the next occasion. This might even ensure that some of the reflections stimulated continue between the consultations. Frequently, the most useful work takes place when the clinician is not present – 'real life' takes over. In this way patients can only give *themselves* the credit for making connections and for working something out. It is also possible for patients to take home the drawing and to share it with a close family member. This also provides continuity, so that the work initiated in the consultation carries on afterwards.

Next please . . .

Ms C, a single woman in her mid-thirties, came to consult her GP because she felt depressed following a hysterectomy for fibroids. She talked about losing her womb and also about not being able to have any children and what that meant to her own image of being a woman. Whilst these were all acknowledged as possible factors accounting for her current depression, Ms C indicated that there was something else she wanted to talk about. Direct questioning was unsuccessful, and when uncertain about where to go next, the GP introduced the Family Circles Method.

The doctor enquired about the circles and remarked that mother seemed to be very big whereas father was somewhat small. After some thought she said that he was in fact her step-father. The GP asked what it was like being brought up by him and Ms C revealed that she had drawn him small and distant from herself and her mother as she wanted to forget about him. Without any further probing she said that he had sexually abused her for years. The operation had brought back these memories vividly, particularly as she stayed with her parents for the first time in 10 years when convalescing. The GP asked her how she felt about telling him all that and she replied that she was very relieved as she had never told a single person about what happened. A further appointment was made at the patient's request for the following week and she told her doctor that she felt better for having told someone about her past experiences. The possibility of more specialist help was discussed, but Ms C declined. During the following year she attended the surgery several times, mostly with ordinary physical ailments. She was generally functioning well and her depression had not returned.

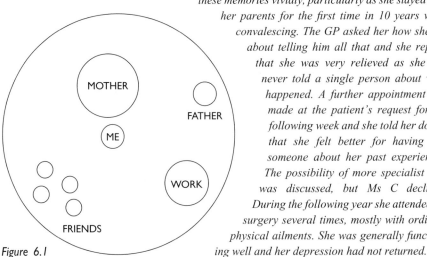

Figure 6.1

Next please . . .

A 38-year-old woman, Mrs D, had attended repeatedly at the surgery complaining about symptoms of anxiety and being depressed. The genogram revealed that she was a single mother with an adolescent daughter. She was worried about her daughter who she suspected was taking drugs. In addition, Mrs D seemed unduly preoccupied with her daughter's awakening sexuality and as her general mental state remained unchanged, the practice counsellor decided to try the Circles technique. The enquiry soon focused on the person drawn outside the large circle. Mrs D referred to him as a 'possible' friend and the conversation then turned to practical steps as to how to turn this person into a 'real' friend if that was what she wanted. Mrs D worked out some concrete moves she needed to make, whilst at the same time exploring the impact this might have on the relation-ship with her daughter. She soon felt less anxious and generally more positive. A year later she had married this 'possible' friend.

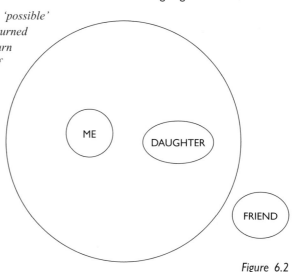

Figure 6.2

Next please ...

A 55-year-old man, Mr W, consulted his primary care team because of serious sleeping prob-lems. He also said that he had to have 'lots of booze' to get some sleep. He acknowledged that he often felt quite low. The practice nurse knew that he had two teenage children and that his wife had died a few years before from a malignant tumour. In the course of this consultation the practice nurse asked him to draw circles. He put himself in the centre with the family neatly grouped around him. Right at the top were the maternal grandparents and the far bottom right-hand corner a woman. It then transpired that the woman was his lover, a Catholic who hap-pened to be married. Mr W said he felt stuck because she wouldn't divorce and he felt guilty, being an active (Protestant) church member and coming from a fairly religious family (as rep-resented by the grandparents in the circles). Looking at all this from the outside enabled Mr W to see his life and belief systems in perspective. He started talking about the pros and cons of staying in the relationship with a married woman from what he perceived to be a different faith.

He thought about all the responses from his family of origin if they found out about his secret relationship. The drawing also showed that his priest was very important to him. He thought he needed to talk to the priest as a first step.

The practice nurse saw Mr W a few weeks later. He told her that he had made a decision following the previous consul-tation. He could see he was caught up in too many moral and real conflicts and that he needed to end the relationship. He reported that since making that decision his sleeping pattern had begun to get better and that he no longer required excess amounts of alcohol to 'put me out'.

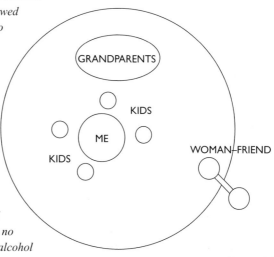

Figure 6.3

Next please . . .

Mr K, age 64, a school teacher about to retire, repeatedly presented with diffuse head and back pains. The genogram revealed nothing surprising, but when Mr K drew the circles, he was very surprised by the size and spatial centrality of one of the circles. This circle, it emerged, represented his work. Mr K laughed and talked about being in need of a 'shrink'. When encouraged to think about how he himself could shrink the monster's size, he came up with quite a few practical solutions. Further consultations focused increasingly less on his physical pains. Instead, he started thinking about the effects of retirement on his relationship with his wife and children.

Figure 6.4

Next please . . .

Mr S, a 40-year-old man originally from Bangladesh, had consulted his primary care team for months with what he described as a 'stabbing heart pain'. After many rounds of different investigations, no physical causes for the recurring pain were found. Mr S did not like the GP's suggestion that he might be depressed or worried – he insisted that his problems were physical. The GP, in despair, asked the practice counsellor to take on Mr S, who told the counsellor that he was 'not mad'. The counsellor replied that he accepted that there was something wrong with Mr S's heart and that it would help to know more about it. He drew a big heart on a piece of paper and asked Mr S to put all the people and all the worries he had inside the outline of the heart drawing. Mr S looked puzzled, but obliged. Soon the picture was

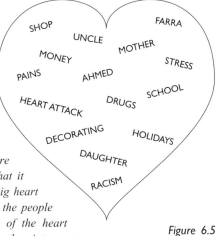

Figure 6.5

filled with many worries and some people. It was literally impossible to stop Mr S talking about each of the worries – as his heart was literally flowing over. He returned for four more sessions and there were no further consultations about his heart pains with any member of the primary care team subsequently.

Next please . . .

Ms T had had two children fostered, as they were born when she was young and she had no support from her alcoholic mother. The children had different fathers and the health visitor (HV) often thought that the social services department had written off Ms T as a poor mother forever. Ms T was pregnant again. Relationships had become strained all round. She was not very bright but had a resilient quality about her that made the HV persist with drawing a family circle. Ms T refused to hold the pen because she couldn't write, but she gave instructions that her new boyfriend and his parents were in the middle with her two fostered children in the circle and the baby in the middle of the new family. She put the HV very close to her, as was the GP whom she saw for monitoring of her asthma. She put the social worker (SW) outside of the circle, saying emphatically that the SW would have drawn herself inside the circle next to Ms T and between her and the baby. The HV asked: 'What would have to happen for you to be able to keep the social worker outside the circle? Who do you need to help you make this happen? What can they say or do?' Together they worked out a list of different behaviours that the SW would need to see: Ms T bonding with the new baby, responding in a less hot-headed way with the SW, and her new 'in-laws' being able to join the core group as they were likely to be a real asset to her.

Figure 6.6

Ms T often referred to this circle as being a pivotal moment. She saw what she had to do. She also felt empowered because she was able to remove the SW from her family in her imagination and see what she had to do to keep her out. She also saw the value of her new family. The HV saw the importance of her maternal granny, whom Ms T had never talked about but who had given Ms T an example of good mothering to follow. Ms T also talked about keeping her mother (living with a schedule one offender) clearly on the edge of the circle to keep her new child safe.

Next please ... the primary care team as patient

A part-time woman doctor decided to talk to the practice psychologist as she felt that she was being pushed out by the practice since the arrival of a new younger full-time doctor. The psychologist helped her by drawing a family circle to look at the shifting pattern of relationships caused by a new arrival and the work that the practice needed to do to negotiate this transition. He then asked the following questions:

- 'Out of the present team, who joined the practice first?'
- 'Who next?'
- 'Who next?'
- 'How have relationships altered with each addition to the team?'
- 'Do you include district nurses, health visitors and community psychiatric nurses in or outside the circle?'

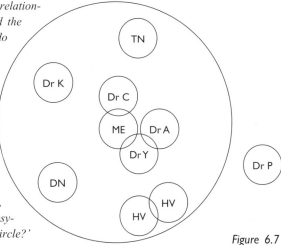

Figure 6.7

- *'How do relationships change when someone leaves the team?'*
- *'If the practice manager and the GPs have several meetings together and get closer in the circle what happens to relationships with the nurses and receptionists?'*
- *'Are there any people who have left the team who should be included on the map?'*
- *'What different patterns of relationship are there to part-time and full-time people working in the practice?'*

Simultaneous family circle drawings

It is possible for various family members to do their family circle drawings simultaneously. This applies to couples as much as to families with children. Young children (who can probably do this from the age of 3 upwards) rarely stick to circles but nevertheless provide interesting images and information that often come as major surprises to their parents. The instruction given is very similar to the one described above, only adding that the family members might want to look at each other's drawings together afterwards. Once everyone has completed their circles, the clinician can ask who would like to start. Discussing the circles is different in that other family members are present and very likely to comment on what is being said. Not infrequently heated discussions ensue, with partners or other family members challenging one another about their respective perceptions of family relationships. Given that in many families beliefs about various issues are never really examined, the Family Circles Method has enormous potential to explode such family myths in a very brief time.

It is also possible to ask two family members to imagine the circles their partner (or parent/child) might draw and then encourage them to do so. If each draws the imagined family life space and relationships of the other, these accounts can then be thought about together. This can provide fascinating insights for each family member, examining their assumptions and receiving feedback.

Working with the whole family

There is another way in which family circles can be used. A whole family – or indeed a couple – can be asked to do this, but only on the same large piece of paper. Doing such a family picture requires a lot of communication and discussion; it also requires compromises and decision making. And it can be a lot of fun – and chaos.

The Family Circles Method enables patients to visualise the way in which different parts of their lives and families are connected. It brings home the point that if one thing changes, other areas of life have to change as well, with ripple effects all round. Significant relationships and support systems can be identified and the implications of change considered. Ironically, in this way the Family Circles Method helps people to come unstuck and not to continue going round and round in circles.

Authors' enthusiasm warning (see also Chapter 12)

In this chapter and elsewhere we have included many clinical examples. These often exemplify interventions, questions, genograms, circles, which 'work' – where change occurs and where there is the 'Ah-ha!' moment. We have done this because we want you to try these things, we want you to be excited and intrigued enough to do something different! But of course, particularly within the very limited time frames we operate under, it will not always be like this. You may try out a circle only to find you have not asked more than one interesting question before the tyranny of time or red diary dates flashing on the computer or looks of blankness on your patients' face steals your bravery and you lapse back into: 'Well, perhaps we should change the antidepressant?'

Well, don't worry, it is like that for us too! Sometimes there are no magic connections, no giant leaps. It is small faltering steps. Lots of people and lots of situations are not amenable to great change. But don't give up, just try it again sometime when you have the headspace to experiment again.

Your own family circle

1   Draw your own family circle as you see it now. Get a friend or colleague to do the same. Interview each other about your drawings. Avoid being too 'clever' – ask questions, do not speculate or project your own ideas onto the drawing. Make a note of questions that you find particularly difficult or useful. Ask your friend what he or she found useful.

2   Now do the same again, but draw the circles in the way you each would like your lives to be in a year's time. Discuss the differences and speculate about what simple steps you could each take to make it happen.

3   Ask the next patient with mild depression or recurrent psychosomatic symptoms to draw their family circle and put the illness in the picture.

4   Draw a family circle for your primary health care team. How do you imagine other team members would draw their views of the team? What three questions could you raise for potential discussion within the team?

Family transitions 7

This chapter covers:
○ Family phases and transition points
○ Family life cycles

So far we have introduced the main ideas of systemic work, situated this work in multiple contexts, and interested you (we hope) in several ways of generating new perspectives on the person within their family context. These have included the asking of circular and reflexive questions, genograms and family circles. All this time we have been encouraging you to develop curiosity as to what 'may be going on' for an individual within his or her context. It is helpful while you are trying to generate new hypotheses to have frameworks to draw upon. These frameworks are not facts about families, they are constructions which, like all stereotypes, have usefulness and limitations. One such framework is the notion of family phases or life cycle stages.

Every family goes through different phases in its life and each new phase presents a challenge to its organisation and equilibrium. When a first-born baby enters the world, her mum's dad overnight becomes grandad, his daughter suddenly a mother and the mother-in-law is now a freshly baked granny! Not only is each family member presented with a new role, but the family as a whole also enters a transition in its development.

 The family life cycle

The concept of the family life cycle (Carter and McGoldrick 1989), describing a family passing through various stages of development and change, is a valuable idea, although there is no consensus about how many stages should be recognised, particularly given the enormous variation in different cultures and the culturally mediated views of the 'self' and 'individuation'. The word 'transition' is useful to hold in mind as change requires emotional and practical tasks to be done.

This requires plenty of adjustments to be made. Three if not four different generations will need to accommodate to life cycle transitions simultaneously. For some, these accommodations may be imperceptibly small, for others incalculably large. As families move through the various phases, so do their individual members, inventing and re-negotiating their relationships with parents, spouses, siblings and others. New family members join through birth, adoption, courting or marriage, and leave by separation, divorce or death – if then! Even if people have left physically, they can still remain very much present – even if only as 'ghosts' in their families' lives, although urns and graves and remembered relatives still occupy physical spaces in the lives of many living families.

These life cycle stage patterns present with often predictable problems and common presentations in primary care settings. An awareness of the family life cycle phases and their potential crisis points allows clinicians to generate hypotheses. They also offer opportunities for preventive action. Antenatal classes, menopause clinics and specific counselling projects exist in many services. Knowledge of developmental family issues leads to anticipatory guidance about the challenges to be faced, if combined with an understanding of the family's resources and successes in managing previous life cycle stages.

Symptoms as a sign of pressure at the transition points

Family stress often occurs at *transition points* from one stage of the family's life cycle to another and symptoms are most likely to appear when there is a disruption in the unfolding cycle, or if a family is going through two or three transitions at once. Remember how keen we were for you to note down dates when you did the family trees in Chapter 5? It was for this reason – to spot the multiple or failed transitions. For example, early marital problems may reflect a spouse's difficulties in separating from their family of origin, and this will be compounded if one of their parents develops a chronic illness and needs additional care.

There is huge variation in how family life cycles evolve, with culture playing a major role. There are no 'right' or 'wrong' ways of negotiating the journey as different cultures have different rites of passage. Moreover, even in the same culture we find enormous variations, based on family composition, class differences, gender assumptions, changing social mores, economic realities and other factors. The concept of the family life cycle can provide useful clinical guidance, but only if it is critically examined and modified according to the contexts to which it is applied.

For growth and maturation to continue in families, each life cycle stage needs to be negotiated. Success or failure to do so are governed by how preceding phases have been managed. It is at the point when the family is unable to adapt to a new situation that one of its members may become symptomatic and present to his or her primary care team. In order to arrive at a new understanding of a patient's complaints, it can be useful to explore recent transitions in the family's life cycle.

Old experiences tend to resonate with new events, such as the birth of a child. Using the framework of the family life cycle can help to put these stories into a historical context and address them in the present. In the above case example it helped to prevent further distress, not only for the patient, but for the family as a whole.

Next please . . .

Mr J consulted his GP repeatedly over diffuse chest and abdominal pains. After a number of inves-
tigations, no organic causes were found for the seemingly mild complaints. When asked in more
detail about the history of the complaints, Mr J revealed that the symptoms had started some three
months ago, shortly after the birth of his first child. When asked what effect this important life
event had had on him, he responded first by saying how happy and fulfilled it had made him.

The GP later asked whether the birth of the baby had also had some 'unwanted side effects'.
(Note what an effective way of gently probing, while not disqualifying his earlier remark, this is.)
Mr J hesitated before he replied that this had 'left me feeling displaced'. He added that he had not
spoken about this to his wife because 'that would make me seem a bit childish. I am not the jeal-
ous type'. Asked whether he thought that there might be a connection between his somatic com-
plaints and the birth of his son, Mr J gasped and said: 'My dad died when I was a baby . . . they
say it was from a heart attack.' The GP asked whether his wife knew about this and
what her response might be if Mr J talked about the possible connection between his present com-
plaints and past experience. Mr J thought it might be a way forward and he returned for
a follow-up consultation two weeks later, feeling much better – both physically and emotionally.

In the following section we shall examine a number of different family life cycle
stages and describe common issues that may arise during these stages and which
may be seen in primary care settings. It is quite arbitrary at which point we enter
the cycle – or circle. So why not start with forming a twosome: 'boy meets boy'
or 'boy meets girl' , or 'girl meets girl' – or is it the other way round?

Next please . . .

Bill, 55, and John, 41, had lived together for 10 years. To their friends they were a happy and
committed couple. Bill's parents were dead, but John's parents were alive and well – and very
Catholic. The idea that their son could be gay seemed unthinkable. John was well aware of that,
hiding his relationship with Bill from them successfully for almost a decade. Living in Ireland
the parents would come over to southern England once a year, forcing Bill and John to put up
a charade: Bill became the 'flatmate', with John camping in the spare room and a few pieces
of furniture being moved about strategically. It was when the parents were no longer fooled by
this performance that one day John saw his GP because of anxiety symptoms.

Becoming a couple

When two adults decide to live together and to form a partnership, both need to
start negotiating a great range of issues. These include how much time to spend
together, where to live, when to sleep, have sex, eat and argue; when and where
to work, how to have holidays and who should read the paper first – and whether
it needs to be ironed after *he* has read it .... . Decisions with regard to finances,
seeing friends and doing the washing-up are no longer determined individually but
jointly. Each partner may have inherited some recipes and tips for survival from
their respective families of origin, but the couple will have to decide which of the
baggage from the past will need to be dumped in order to make a start that suits
them both, and of course also both hold on determinedly to behaviours it feels too
risky to lose.

Life cycle stages

Study the list of family life cycle stages and problems (Table 7.1).

1   Think about which phase you think you (and your family) are in – and how this schema 'fits'. Any familiar changes or problems?
2   Look at the 'common presenting problems' column and go over all the patients you've seen today. How many presented with these problems or symptoms? What do you know about their life cycle phases?
3   Now think about the limitations of the table. Which cultures does it not fit? What might be the dangers of promoting Eurocentric models?
4   Now photocopy the table and keep it with all your guidelines and protocols on – or under – your office desk. No, on second thoughts, keep it somewhere you might actually use it to generate some more ideas!

Extended families have many ways of accepting or rejecting the partner of their beloved grown-up 'child'. And these 'children' have their own ways of inviting in – or excluding – their own parents and other significant members of the family. It is hardly surprising that this is a time for potential tension that may test each partner's loyalties. Those who have found marriage the only way of escaping from their families of origin may continue to remain very involved emotionally with their families even after they have ostensibly formed a twosome. A mixture of guilt and resentment often leads to confrontations between the spouses, with a request for the in-laws to stop 'interfering'. Other couples cut off their parents or other members of their family of origin – again often with rather mixed feelings. However, even putting thousands of miles and an ocean between themselves and their parents may not bring about the separation some may have hoped for.

Most couples test what they have learned in their respective families of origin: in this way they quickly discover that it is possible to transfer fights one used to have with one's parents directly to the partner. Conversely there is no reason why one should not replicate positive experiences and many partners succeed in selecting those recipes they have tasted as being successful in their respective family of origin. Yet, there may well be some conflict as to which partner's family scripts should be used in the present relationship. Some individuals feel so over-connected with their families of origin that they may exclude their other half from that important part of their life, thereby fostering exclusive relationships which are bound to produce problems sooner or later. It could be said that such adults appear to be 'married' to their parents rather than to their spouses. This can sometimes lead to there being six people in the marital bed rather than just two! And there are those so-called 'grown-ups' who choose partners to handle their families for them, a solution that may work initially, but often creates plenty of problems in the long term, with the partner getting increasingly embroiled in adverse family dynamics.

Table 7.1 'Western' family life cycle phases and problems

Phase	Task	Required family changes	Common presenting problems
Becoming a couple	Commitment to each other and extended families	Agreeing roles and goals, negotiating intimacy, realigning relationships inside and outside family	Sexual problems, infertility, headaches, chest or back pains
Becoming parents	Integrating new member	Adjusting twosome to threesome, negotiating parental roles: wife, woman and/or mother? Man, husband, father? Restricting social life	Crying, feeding and sleeping problems, 'baby blues', couple tension and affairs, child neglect and abuse
Growing children	Nurturing	Balancing home and outside world demands, practising child–parent separations	Out-of-control child behaviours, enuresis, soiling, tics, jealousy and sibling fights, abdominal pain
Conquering adolescence	Establishing new boundaries	Balancing control versus independence, permitting to move in and out of family, encouraging difference and experimentation	Staying out late, running away, school refusal and truancy, eating disorders, domestic violence, drug and alcohol issues, parasuicide
Launching children	Leaving and letting go	Filling 'empty nest', parents establish new relationship with one another – and the home leaver, separation and independence	Psychotic or eccentric behaviour of home leaver, marital problems, mid-life crisis
The family in later life	Coping with loss and changing roles	Managing illness and death of (grand)parents, growing into grandparental roles, adjusting to widow-hood	Bereavement and prolonged grief reaction, depression, dementia, physical illness and concordance problems

Religious and cultural conventions are often of great significance. In families which have migrated from an Eastern to a Western culture, we can see conflicts arising when the parental expectations of marriage and kinship conflict with those their offspring encounter in the host culture. For example, if the expectation of having their marriage arranged by the parents is frustrated by the grown-up children, we are likely to see conflicts that may well manifest themselves in physical symptoms – either in one of the young partners or in the disappointed parent. Families can work hard at trying to block seemingly inappropriate liaisons, whether across racial or class barriers or whether for religious or lifestyle reasons, or to do with strong views in relation to homosexual relationships. Whether the next generation is prepared to put up with the expectations or prescriptions from their elders is another matter: stoic acceptance or violent rejection of parental expectations can be equally troublesome for the young person and result in problematic behaviour all round.

Common presentations in primary care during this stage of the life cycle include sexual problems, infertility and non-specific somatic complaints.

Next please ...

Farra's marriage had been arranged by her parents. She had seemed happy with their choice of husband. He was 25 years older and a distinguished member of the community. It was three years into the marriage that both consulted their GP because of what they called 'infertility' problems. The second consultation revealed that the marriage had not been consummated. Dr K felt quite out of her depth dealing with this issue. Her first inspiration was to invite the midwife for the next consultation. Both noticed that Ali, the husband, felt very uncomfortable. The next inspiration was to ask one of their male doctor colleagues to 'have a word' with Ali. The next step was to invite the Imam to have an all-male conversation. Farra seemed to feel all right about it, but Dr K and the midwife did not. Eight weeks later Farra announced that she was pregnant. We will never know what really happened.

Becoming parents

The change from a twosome to a threesome can not only shake the equilibrium in the couple but also in the families of origin. Privacy and intimacy move into the background, for the time being, often much to the annoyance of at least one if not both partners. The new baby often heralds the return of the in-laws, with all its positive and problematic aspects. Too much help can be perceived as being a problem. Grandparental financial input can carry the implication that this gives permission for them to advise if not dictate 'what's best for everyone'. When the threesome is a result of assisted fertilisation or through fostering or adoption, then a different, and perhaps less predictable set of behaviours ensues. How do grandparents relate to babies that are not blood relatives, or partners or couples to children with no genetic connections?

Repeated presentation of the baby at the surgery for very minor complaints can be a sign that a young family is unable to cope with the transitions required to adapt to this new phase in its life cycle. Crying, feeding and sleeping problems are more than familiar to every member of the primary care team. Mother may complain about feeling 'low' and, on further exploration, reveals that she feels unattractive and unsupported by her husband who claims that he needs his sleep badly to be able to keep his job. The more he withdraws, the more his wife gets exhausted – and the more the husband feels that his wife is no longer interested in him. This is a time when an affair seems the 'only solution' for quite a few men. (Women get their turn later, when they have recovered from child-rearing, as you will see! But remember, all of you diversity-sensitive people, who are shifting uncomfortably in your reading chairs, all this is only one set of stories about what may happen. There are lots of other possibilities – it is just about opening up your 'thought channels' about what may be happening!)

When working with young families in primary care, it is important to pick up any warning signs early on. It is crucial that both parents are seen together as there is a great likelihood that they affect one another intensely – and the baby. Clinicians can facilitate the couple to talk to each other about how to resolve specific issues (see Chapter 9), usually to do with managing the baby, and the strains on the couple's relationship as the result of having become a threesome. Becoming parents inevitably puts a lot of strain on couples and it is therefore not surprising to learn that a very high proportion of relationships or marriages break up within a year of the first child being born. Supporting parents at this stage can prevent couples from separating. It often needs a team approach; 10 minutes may be enough to find out the problems and to assess their urgency, but it will not be enough to resolve them.

Growing children

As babies get older they become toddlers, they enter school and they never stop making seemingly endless demands on their parents: the road from the 'terrible twos' to the 'vile teenager' is paved with many pleasures – and pains. At the beginning of this long and generally rewarding journey parents will be preoccupied with 'taming the monster'. This involves teaching the toddler to eat the 'right' food at the 'right' time, to go to bed at the 'right' time, to say the 'right' things at the 'right' time, to put their excrements in the 'right' place – and so on. Is it a surprise that these little children turn into monsters, having to comply with all the unreasonable demands of their controlling parents? One thing all toddlers seem to have in common is that they quickly become world champions at defeating their parents. Moreover, they also seem to have magic powers to make their parents disagree with one another as to what is the 'right' thing to do.

Next please . . .

Laura (28) presented to the midwife pregnant for the first time. The midwife had read the records and seen that Laura had had counselling for marital and sexual difficulties with the practice psychologist. She had had a very difficult relationship with her mother who could not be expected to be helpful after the birth. Laura had also been on antidepressants. The midwife decided that she needed to meet with the psychologist and health visitor to discuss the issues of preventing breakdown in the couple's relationship and to manage a possibly difficult delivery because of vaginismus. The team developed a shared understanding of the need for thinking about the individuals, the three new dyadic relationships, and the extended family. They looked carefully at the boundaries of their respective roles and how they could communicate concerns. They agreed an action plan with Laura and her husband Mike. Over the next two weeks, both Laura and Mike were to book daily 'appointments', lasting 10 minutes, with one another. During these times each had five

A couple of exercises

Here are a couple of exercises you might like to try. Yes! we know, we give you lots of exercises and you may want to ignore them and just get on with the good read, but remember – doing the exercise puts the learning in the bit of your brain with a longer half-life!

1 Choose two patients on today's list (or make the decision to think about two people who you see tomorrow) and try to figure out as much as you can about where they may be in the life cycle. What is the nearest transition they have been through or are to come to? Note any interesting thoughts about what is happening and whether it could have any connection with today's presentation.

2 Have a think about what life cycle stage you are at. What was the last transition and what is the next to come? Think about what, if anything, has been significant about these transitions and any connections with your own or other people's health. As an extra, try to imagine what your particular stage might be like if you were in a different sort of relationship, gay or straight, with biological or adoptive children or the child of adoptive parents, etc. What changes and what are some of the more universal issues that need to be negotiated and navigated?

minutes to talk about any worries or concerns, with the other being merely in a listening position. At the end of the 'appointment' Laura and Mike should not talk for another 10 minutes, but could go about their respective businesses.

When she next saw the midwife, Laura said that for the first time in the relationship she felt that her husband had been listening to her. Mike was also positive about understanding his wife better – though he said that he had found it difficult to talk for five minutes . . . .

The most frequent presentation in primary care with families feeling trapped in this particular phase of the life cycle are parental exhaustion (and anger) and 'out-of-control' behaviours in children. Frequently the parents do not agree on how to handle their toddler's outbursts, with one parent characteristically being 'too soft' and the other inevitably 'too harsh'. Soiling, enuresis, sleeping between the parents in the marital bed (or, a common variation, the toddler sleeping with mother in the marital bed and father sleeping in the toddler's bed next door), jealousy and continuous fighting between siblings – these are all too familiar scenarios in this family phase.

Whether they are seen as problems and by whom is, of course, one of the issues. Clinicians, as always, need to be sensitive to what the participants perceive as problems, not what they, as clinicians (but also often parents) hear as problems. 'Is this the way you would like it to be, Lynsdey/Francis/Farooq?'

Providing appropriate care at this stage of the life cycle, using the wider teams attached to primary care can be bewildering. Does this mum need a health visitor or a community psychiatric nurse for herself, or her GP to provide antidepressants?

Who takes the lead for maternal mental health? If the father is having problems, whom should he see?

Next please ...

Mr R went to his GP looking sheepish and embarrassed. He asked for some help to control his anger as he had 'knocked the Misses about a bit'. She had threatened to leave him and take their 2-year-old daughter with her. The GP felt anxious about the child protection implications of this presentation, as Mr R had two convictions for assault. The GP considered the following interventions, informed by a life cycle perspective, and how these could be done in 10-minute consultations:

* *Looking at the family patterns with a genogram (Mr R's father had left when he was 2)*
* *Helping the family to develop 'keeping themselves safe strategies' (see Chapter 9)*
* *Talking about the ingredients of good fathering and what Mr R did do well despite his upbringing – attending to strengths*
* *Strengthening the couple's identity as a couple and not just as parents*
* *Negotiating permission to talk to Mr R's partner and check out safety issues*
* *Sharing anxieties with other team members.*

Conquering adolescence

To many parents – and a considerable number of clinicians – adolescence is not just a life cycle stage but an illness in its own right! Eating, money, sex, friends, school, God(s) – almost anything can become problematic. Adolescents go through plenty of open and secret identity crises and they can drag their families up and down through prolonged periods of stress. Everything seems to be in flux, oscillating between demands for autonomy and reproaches over not being cared for enough. Parents fluctuate between encouraging their young person to be independent and at the same time being over-controlling: one minute they ask their teenager to 'clear out and never come back again', only to be followed moments later by pleading with the youngster to 'come back home again'. The 'four-year age gap' is the phenomenon of parents perceiving their child as being two years younger than he or she actually is, while the child feels at least two years older than the actual biological age. One of the tasks clinicians often face is to attempt to decrease this virtual age gap between the generations, so that more mutual understanding can take place.

Parents sometimes attend together, sometimes alone, sometimes they start somewhere else but end up complaining bitterly about their offspring's provocative and irresponsible behaviours which threaten to break up the family. Problems include: drug taking, truancy, violence, general disruptiveness at school and at home, demonstrative sexual behaviour, self-neglect and self-harming, eating disorders, mixing in bad company and so on. It is rare that the teenager in question accompanies the parents to the surgery which seems to underline further the parents' claim that their son or daughter is beyond control. The parents themselves may present with physical or emotional symptoms of stress, whether headaches or backaches, anxiety states or depression. Of course, all these things are familiar and obvious when you know they are happening. The point, of course, is picking up these presentations when you did not know that your patient had a gothic teenager living in a dark purple room with the blinds down and a curious smell emanating from under the door, or a mini-skirted, alcopop-drinking, E-popping 13-year-old starting to argue with your patient's new boyfriend about when she should be back home each night! That's when the third consultation about periods or headaches or insomnia begins to make more sense.

Next please ...

John (16) presented with his mother complaining of headaches for two months and a worry that he felt so awful that he didn't think he could take his mock exams. He was very anxious and had frequent episodes of hyperventilating. His mother was anxious about what she should be saying as, in her view, he was old enough to come to the doctor on his own. She mentioned that he had started drinking a bit more than she would like him to. After some of the parental anxieties had begun to settle down and his mother no longer believed he was dying of a brain tumour, the following questions, addressed to John, were useful in providing a new focus:

- *'Who else in your family is highly strung?'*
- *'How do other members of the family cope with tensions?'*
- *'What are the advantages and disadvantages of being a highly strung person?'*
- *'Just thinking of being anxious in the future, one of the ways that young men manage anxiety, stress and worries is to drink alcohol, but they often aren't aware of why they are drinking so the drinking becomes a problem in its own right. What do you think about that?'*
- *'Now you know about anxiety, how might you monitor the reasons for how much you might be drinking?'*
- *'Having had this discussion today with your mum listening would you want her to notice your anxiety levels or do you want to do your own noticing and taking care of yourself?'*
- *'How old will you be when you will do most of the worrying for yourself?'*

It can be hard to strike the balance of respecting the parents' views and giving the young person a sense of being heard and respected in their own right. We don't always get it right.

Launching children

The 'empty nest' is a prospect some families cherish as it heralds a time of more freedom, with the possibility of taking up long neglected hobbies or pursuing new interests. Other families dread this phase and try to put it off, worrying about how to fill the space(s) vacated by the grown-up 'child'. If the parents still live together, then it is often a time to re-evaluate their couple relationship: they may consider 'getting married again' or separating. Often the parents face simultaneous demands both from their grown children as well as from their own parents. This curious position between generations has earned people going through this stage the label the 'sandwich' generation, pressed by the needs of the young who may still be financially and emotionally dependent on them whilst at the same time recruited by the newly dependent elderly. Young people growing apart from their families are led to find out more about themselves, in what ways they are similar to or different from their parents and sibs, which family expectations they are willing to meet and which not. It is a time for experiments with peer relationships, relating to a work context, maybe facing unemployment and financial hardship. On the other hand, young people sometimes flex their muscles and profess total independence, but are soon scared of their own courage (Haley 1979).

In primary care, clinicians often find themselves having to deal with a suddenly bereaved parent – even though nobody has actually died. It can also be the 'retired' parents' marriage which is presented as the problem. This is a time when divorces tend to happen more frequently, often coinciding with the menopause. Mental and physical fatigue, sexual inadequacy, job stress, alcohol and nicotine abuse are common presentations at this time. The prospect of retirement may raise additional fears, particularly about filling the empty spaces.

Next please . . .

Mrs B had seen her GP because of several months of depression. One antidepressant had failed, another one followed with an equal lack of success. A new antidepressant had just been introduced to an already saturated market – should Dr L try this one out next? Before contemplating doing so, he asked Mrs B to draw some family circles (see Chapter 6). She drew herself in the middle of an otherwise empty 'life' circle, placing two other big circles far away from her. These turned out to be her two children who had left home. When asked about how the picture would have looked like prior to their departure, she drew a rich pattern of circles all around her. When requested to look at the first picture and put 'depression' in, she smiled and said: 'I guess that's what's taken the place of my children.' Her GP then got her to consider how else she could fill the space her children had vacated. This was the beginning of replacing 'depression' with more positive relationships and activities, rendering further antidepressants unnecessary.

The family in later life

Over time the family circle is enlarged by new partners and grandchildren. It is intrinsic in the concept of the family life cycle that many of the phases happen simultaneously: as some members get older, others enter the family as babies. As parts of the family machinery get rejuvenated, other parts get rusty. In most families there come times when there is a specific preoccupation with the older members, their physical state and their open or veiled requests for help. It is a time when primary care workers see their patients presenting with physical illness, such as angina, arthritis and diabetes. Clinicians attend not only to the various physical ailments, but also to how their patients emotionally handle their deteriorating health. Furthermore, old(er) age is a time of major losses: job, friends, spouse and other relatives, money, status, mental faculties and so on. Some elderly patients may, knowingly or unknowingly, use physical illness or symptoms to draw in their relatives, with emerging resentment and guilt on everyone's part, including physical or emotional symptoms in the younger generation. Often it is the relatives or carers who need major help as they may be overburdened with anxiety or 'carer depression', unable to meet the many demands made upon them (Asen 2001).

There are many myths surrounding the ageing process, for instance that people get more rigid and less capable of change as they age. In fact, talking treatments can work well as the older adult has much more life experience and resilience to draw on. Counselling services for this age group have to change their focus as retirement often throws an elderly person back into past traumas. People in their sixties and seventies now may get nightmares about being separated from their families by evacuation during the Second World War and may need more attachment tuned ways of working. For people in their eighties, wartime experiences can come alive, not infrequently triggered by physical illness, with flashbacks and related anxiety symptoms emerging.

Next please . . .

A 77-year-old woman, retired at 75, has seldom visited the doctor. She then developed arthritis and needed a knee replacement. After the operation she became profoundly depressed. Her GP saw her on five separate occasions for brief consultations and learned that she had been a teenager during the Second World War, being the youngest of six children. The war for her had meant: being bombed out of the family home, a brother becoming schizophrenic, her sister's fiancé being killed in action, her father being killed on his bicycle in the black-out, a brother being injured at work and herself being admitted to a sanatorium with TB. She seemed to have coped with this succession of traumas by being cheerful and keeping busy. She pursued a career in social reform to make life better for others. Until her retirement she had never had a time of inactivity and convalescence and, not surprisingly she found the struggle of coping with this aspect of ageing unbearable. However, during the course of these 10-minute consultations she connected past with present, grieving about her losses and remembering very vividly her hospitalisation as a teenager. She brought her husband to the consultations – he had not known about the detail of his wife's traumatic experiences. She found it was a relief to get him involved in her past life and he gave her strength to become mobilised again.

Perceptions of ageing

Consider the following:

- On a scale of 0–10 with 0 = not at all likely and 10 = very likely, how rigid and set in their ways do you think elderly people are?
- On the same scale, how likely do you think it is that they can be worked with therapeutically – and change?
- What experiences led you to arrive at these figures?
- On a scale of 0–10, how likely are you to change your perceptions or prejudices as you get older? Oh, and by the way, how old are you?

Assessing, reflecting and connecting

This chapter covers:
- Systemic assessments along nine different dimensions
- The importance of reflecting
- The usefulness of making hypotheses
- How to formulate interventions

Systemic assessment – if it's a good one, it's part of therapeutic change as well

Primary care clinicians have generally been trained to undertake the assessment of a patient first and then, based on the findings, to devise a treatment plan. In the field of psychological medicine the process of assessment is often the beginning of treatment or, to put it more systemically, assessment and treatment are inextricably linked: it is impossible to know where one begins and the other ends. For example, we have seen that asking a whole series of circular questions (see Chapter 4) can itself be viewed as an intervention, with the patient becoming increasingly self-reflective, gradually perhaps even questioning his own story about the illness. Such 'interventive interviewing' is often the beginning of the process of change.

In this book we have repeatedly emphasised how questioning the presenting symptom or problem – and the effects it has on others, their responses and the 'dance' around it – opens up new perspectives. The presenting problem is usually a good starting point, but there are many other areas that could benefit from probing further – or from thinking about system(at)ically. It is possible to generate a more general framework of thought and action that one could call 'systemic assessment' – though in primary care that can seem a lengthy title for what one can realistically achieve in 10-minute consultations.

Systemic practitioners have, over the decades, put forward a whole range of different assessment models and we have adapted them for the purposes of this book with, wait for it, nine different dimensions (PPRACTICE, after Christie-Seely 1984)! Although, in practice we cannot, within the time frames and pressures of primary care, afford to undertake lengthy comprehensive systemic assessments, an overall assessment framework can guide the clinician and make it possible to pick out one or two dimensions in each consultation (Table 8.1). If you are stuck you can refer to it and see whether there is an area that you could become curious about

Table 8.1   The nine dimensions of PPRACTICE

System dimension	Description	Clinician's interventions
Problem	The illness itself, nature, duration The result of the illness The meaning of the illness The effect of the illness on the family or community	Listen to problem Highlight effects on everyone in family Enable family members to talk to each other
Problem solving	Identifying the problem Discussing the problem Trying out solutions Discussing the feedback	Enable family members to use their own problem-solving skills
Roles, rules and responsibilities	Sickness role Caring role Provider role Authority Couple, parental, sibling roles and responsibilities Gendered roles Safety responsibilities Role of professionals	Talk about sick person's change of role Consider new roles of each family member Clarify power structure Consider new rules for times of change Address safety issues Convene network meeting
Affect	Close Distant Everyday involvement Emergency responses Coping strategies Management of anger and sadness	Show empathy Enable a variety of feelings to be expressed Find out about family patterns of coping, and expression of emotion Review strategies
Communication	Direct or indirect	Facilitate open and clear communication Challenge conspiracy of silence/unfinished business Challenge covert coalitions or 'triangles'
Time in life cycle	Transitions Effect of illness on transitions	Discuss imminent issues of change for all the family Discuss alternative scenarios
Illness history	Beliefs/fears about illness Patterns of illness over generations Relationships with health professionals Connections with scripts, beliefs and myths	Talk about fears and beliefs and their relationship to past experiences Talk about how to get the best out of services
Community resources	Extended family – strengths and weaknesses Engaged/disengaged with community Social support structures	Identify helpful resources in family and community and how to use them Challenge beliefs about families doing it all or community having to provide it all
Environment	Ethnic origins Religious beliefs Social class Employment and leisure Finance and housing Discrimination	Consider that the family experiences discrimination Consider the effects of poverty and racism Meet with other agencies

and that could inspire your work with a patient, assisting you in formulating hypotheses and perhaps even devising appropriate interventions.

Table 8.1 gives a shorthand version of the different dimensions of a systemic assessment. The text below describes each of the dimensions in more detail. As with many of the ideas and tools in this book you are not meant to do all of this at once. We know how conscientious and self-critical you lot all are! Just dip in and out – use it to stimulate a new idea – not all the time, just when you find yourself drifting into automatic pilot (unless for self-preservation reasons you need to stay in automatic pilot).

P – Presenting problem

Generally each consultation starts with a description of the problem(s). If there is more than one person involved, then there may well be a number of different descriptions. You may find that for the person with an illness, it is its history and the physical or psychological pain that is the problem. For the partner it may be the effect of the illness on the relationship that is most pressing. Systemic clinicians are not only interested in the patient's story of the illness, but also other people's narratives and a general sense of the place of 'the problem' or 'the illness' in the family and wider network. We have already described techniques of questioning the problem in previous chapters, including 'putting the problem in the chair'.

Practising PPRACTICE

- Photocopy this assessment framework table.
- Place it on your office desk or scan into the PC.
- The next time you are stuck in a consultation, just choose one dimension and start thinking about it in relation to a patient and family.
- Another time choose another dimension and do the same.
- Make some brief notes about what you find out.
- Review all your notes a few weeks later.

P – Problem solving

It can be important to find out and assess how the patient, the family and the larger system are generally able to solve – or re-solve – problems. When the family comes up against a problem, do they panic? Does only one person make decisions, with all the others following blindly (and reluctantly), or are several approaches tried? Is there general paralysis and an appeal to professionals? Does the professional system get stimulated into action – or infected by the paralysis?

Problem solving can be divided into a number of distinct stages, adapted from D'Zurilla (1986) among others:

- Identify the problem
- Discuss the problem
- Brainstorm about possible solutions
- Choose and try out one solution
- Discuss the results.

That is the theory – yet, in practice things are not usually that straightforward. For example, a family with a secret, like sexual abuse or domestic violence, may not be able to even identify the problem, let alone discuss it. Another family with a high level of hostility and critical remarks, such as at times of divorce, may be able to identify the problem but not have strategies to sit down and discuss it.

Clinicians can assess a couple's or family's problem-solving skills by asking:

> *How do you, as a family, generally manage or solve problems? Problems such as how to deal with limited finances, who should clear up the mess someone else has made, how to cope with mother's forgetfulness, with husband's back pain, or with teenager's glue sniffing? Or even with mundane problems such as which movie to go to, where to go on holiday?*

This is a first step. If patient or family do not spontaneously come up with some concrete problem, the clinician will ask for examples, and preferably recent ones. It is possible to use the five-stage problem-solving model, with a tight time frame: two minutes on identifying and agreeing on the problem; another two minutes discussing it; another two minutes for brainstorming about possible solutions or strategies – and then making a decision and plan as to how and when to implement it, in another two minutes. The clinician has to be a strict timekeeper! On follow-up, once the solution has been tried, there is then a discussion of what happened and the results. In the light of feedback 'more of the same' solution may be pursued – or modified.

Problem-solving therapy is often talked about in relation to single patients (Mynors-Wallis *et al.* 1995). It is our belief that you are likely to get more successful solutions when you involve more than one person's perspective. One of the problems with people's problem-solving efforts is that they get very wedded to their own solutions. And if these do not work they add to the problem by blaming someone else or simply trying out their preferred solution with more effort. The 'if you don't understand my language I will just say it again while raising my voice' approach! Questions to the individual like: 'What do you think your partner would think of this particular solution?', 'If your daughter was suggesting the solutions not you, what might she say?', 'Is there another solution that others suggest which you are not keen to mention?' may help in the search for better solutions.

R – Roles, rules and responsibilities

An episode of acute illness can reverse roles from one day to the next. For example, if mother is suddenly hospitalised, father may be required to take on child-caring tasks which he has avoided for years. Moreover, in cases of serious acute illness, the medical care system may take over major family roles, often conflicting with parental roles. Hospitalised children in particular have to cope with a new system of rules imposed on them, which may or may not tally with those at home, thus causing additional conflict. Some families find it difficult to compete with the round-the-clock nursing care that hospitals can provide. This may result in the family being tempted to leave an elderly person in hospital or a nursing home for much longer than needed.

Next please ...

Mrs F told the health visitor that her husband was 'always' getting her down and that this made her feel 'tired all the time'. Mr F said that his wife's continuous 'nagging' left him no choice but to respond negatively to her 'endless complaining'. The health visitor spent a few minutes with the couple on identifying the problem as 'constant arguments'. When discussing this, each partner stated that they felt 'misunderstood' by the other. Brainstorming about possible solutions to address the misunderstandings that led to arguments resulted in a number of possible courses of action. Both agreed to experiment with the following:

- *Deciding to have a 'constant argument' at a certain time each day and having to save things up for that time.*
- *Treating each 'constant argument' as though it was a crossword clue with a right answer and to be curious about all possible sides to the story, including the views of friends and family.*
- *Identifying what they used to do when they weren't having 'constant arguments' and to do more of these things.*
- *Remembering how they had solved problems in the past and how others in the family solve problems.*
- *Deciding to have one argument a day in which they try to see the funny side of what they do.*

After a few weeks the health visitor asked them: 'Out of all these possible solutions, which is the one that you think stands the best chance of success? If it is successful how will you be able to repeat it so that it becomes part of a continuing way of getting on? Which solution would be the most difficult for you to try? Which one do you want to experiment with first?'

Assessing roles, rules and responsibilities of different family members – and professionals – can throw new light on how families and other systems manage. Furthermore, it can help them to question how they are managing stress and change.

Dr Homeostat

Whilst it is impossible for clinicians not to play an important role in the early phases of an illness, long-term input can have unwanted side effects. Over-involvement by the clinician may lead to over-dependence, with the family relying heavily on the clinician, as if he or she were the regulator or homeostat of the family. Sometimes it can seem that the clinician has been given an 'honorary family membership'. Wishing to renounce such membership and becoming less available to patient and family results in increasingly more demands being made on 'Dr Homeostat', for example, by a sudden apparent deterioration in the patient's state, seemingly requiring more intensive involvement by the primary care worker(s). Do you recognise this phenomenon? Can you think of a particular family where you might play a bit of this role? How do you get out of this? How about this:

> *I am aware of how much I am involved in the life of your family. I am concerned that my continued input could have less good effects on you: the more I see you, the more you might believe that you cannot handle things by yourselves. And the less you are able to handle things by yourselves, the more I see you. It's like a vicious circle. Perhaps there is a different way of working on this together. Your problems are a challenge but I know you have all sorts of strengths and resources to call on [list some]. I would like to hear from you at our next meeting about the solutions you have been finding for yourselves.*

> *It is very curious but I often find that I can be more helpful to families between crises. I think the reason for this is that when the air is clear, it is easier to discuss and to prepare for the next crisis and then that crisis is much more manageable because of the preparation.*

Next please . . .

Mr G, age 30, has developed reactive arthritis and cannot work. His wife has had to take over the breadwinning responsibility while he struggles with childcare with a 2-year-old and an 8-year-old stepson. They do not have family living nearby though Mrs G has a large network of friends. The 8-year-old has had to grow up and assume roles like carrying in the coal and the wood. He also helps with the shopping, putting bags into the car. Teachers say he is rather disruptive but are managing him. Mr G feels completely demolished by his loss of role and work-based friendship network. Together he and his wife think of ways around this. She knows he is envious of her friends since the arthritis. The 2-year-old seems to have the role of making everyone laugh.

Family structures

Choose a patient and their family and look at how roles and functions in the family are allocated.

*   Who anticipates or experiences role strains?
*   Who takes responsibility for safety issues, such as medication, compliance, anger or violence?
*   What is the power structure in the family?
*   Who makes the decisions in the family?
*   Is it hard for men to do women's caring roles?
*   How do family members agree about doing things differently?
*   What is the role of the helping system?
*   How does it aid or block the family's own sense of responsibility?

You could use this set of questions as an *aide-mémoire* on your desk.

On other occasions you may wish to recognise your role and seek simply to control any escalation in it, negotiating, insisting or settling for a smaller part in the family play.

A – Affect

There are considerable personal and cultural differences in how much emotion people show and how they do this. Expression of affect cannot be simply measured in decibels, millilitres or megabytes. In many cultures, acute severe illness is frequently accompanied by an initial phase of dazed denial, which is then followed by anxiety, hope and fear, and often resentment towards the ill member. It is very important that such a sequence of affective states is acknowledged and that family members are able to talk about these often contradictory feelings. This is especially so if family members are at different stages along the sequence of feelings. You may get a strong sense that under the cheerful feelings bubbling at the surface, there is a profound sadness. You may notice that 'of course I love you dear' is said in a very cross, unloving voice or that family members' body language just do not match the feelings being talked about.

Next please . . .

Mrs J has four children (10–16) who are all struggling with life's demands in one way or another: asthma, headaches, recurrent respiratory infections, exams. She often brings most of them into the surgery for her appointments with a 'Oh, while I'm here with them could I ask you about . . .'. The GP notices that they all look to their mother whenever he asks a question. He knows that they have become a single parent family in the last year after dad moved out to be with another woman. When he asks about how they feel about dad not being there and whether it has any bearing on how they feel, they all intensify their efforts to get mum to answer for them.

Clinician: 'I notice that when I ask questions about difficult feelings, you all turn to your mum like she was a sort of emotional switchboard for the family. I wonder whether mum has

Emotions

Choose a patient and their family and look at how affect and emotions are managed.

- Who is the emotional switchboard of the family?
- Who is most/least able to talk about feelings?
- Are all family members able to express both positive and negative emotions?
- Are there feelings not being openly expressed?
- Can the family provide emotional warmth only at times of crisis but not with everyday issues?

Jot down this set of questions and use them to help remember during the next assessment.

had to carry a lot of responsibility since dad left. I expect there have been lots of difficult feelings, some of you missing him, some cross with him, some pleased that he's not there to tell you off or upset mum. Is it OK for the children to talk about these things?'

C – Communication

'Everything is communication' and 'you cannot *not* communicate' are popular phrases used by communication theorists (Watzlawick *et al.* 1967). True though these statements might be, what are we humble clinicians to make of them in practice? Do we then just observe and assess 'everything'? Where do we begin – and where do we end? Here are a few pragmatic tips for confused clinicians:

- Who talks to whom and who talks for whom?
- Who talks most, who talks least?
- Which topic silences whom?
- Is there a 'switchboard operator' through whom all lines of communication run?
- What are the patterns of interruptions, blocking, side-tracking, mist creating?
- Who gangs up with whom against who – and around what issue?

Any of these observations can be fed back directly to the couple or the family: 'I notice that whenever you talk about this, your husband shrugs his shoulders and interrupts you. What do you think about that? Is it helpful?' or 'I notice that when you talk about your mother, your daughter becomes totally silent and seems to stare into empty space.' These and other observations of communication and meta-communication patterns between family members are, of course, minor interventions in their own right. Drawing attention to what the observing (or observation constructing) clinician 'sees' requires family members to respond – if only in their own heads. In that sense the clinician's intervention is a meta-communication in its own right.

T – Time in life cycle

Connecting the presenting problem, symptom or illness with the patient's position in the life cycle of the family may be a way of understanding more. Acute and chronic illnesses do have different effects on the family at different times in the life cycle and are also more likely to occur at certain points. For example, the young child will be exposed to the risk of infection when entering school; a coronary is most likely at the time of multiple stresses (midlife crisis) and acute illness is more frequent in the frail elderly. However, this is only one dimension – and a rather superficial one. In the previous chapter we have described how life cycle transitions are points of potential and likely crises for individuals, couples and families. Using this frame can help to create a new perspective from which to view a specific problem and the dynamics surrounding it.

I – Illness history

How families view illness varies a great deal, reflecting individual experiences and family narratives, as well as more general social and cultural values and frames. All these, in turn, affect individual and family coping strategies. There are, for instance, parents who get extremely distressed at the slightest sign of their child sickening, always suspecting meningitis or some other potentially fatal illness. What are the past experiences, or stories, that lead to such anxieties, anxieties that other parents simply do not have? How is it that other parents are seemingly oblivious to any sign of distress from their child?

The meanings that families attach to symptoms can be explored by examining each family member's beliefs and fears about illness – and how illness is spread. An exploration of the patterns of health and illness in previous generations can be done with the help of a genogram. It is at times also important to elicit each person's experience of past and present relationships with health professionals.

It is common that each family member's illness story is different, as there will be various preconceptions about the likely causes, course and prognosis of the condition. Is it genetically transmitted? What does that say about us as parents? Is it punishment for some past sins? If the 'storyteller' is a pre-school child, the account may be coloured by the world of fairy tales, inhabited by evil witches, spells and magic cures.

Altschuler (1997) has helpfully summarised systemic ideas and techniques that can be used when exploring the 'illness story'. These include:

Communication and meta-communication

The pioneers of systemic work (Bateson *et al.* 1956, Watzlawick *et al.* 1967) studied and highlighted the influence of communication sequences in families. They concluded that there is a surface level of communication which is qualified by another, higher order level: that of meta-communication. For example, at the surface level there may be a verbal communication (Father: 'I really like your new boyfriend, Jane'), which at a para- or non-verbal level is contradicted (father ignores him, makes hostile noises whenever boyfriend speaks). Furthermore, these pioneers have pointed out that how we make sense of any given communication is also determined by what we want to hear or understand – and by the relationship context within which this communication exchange takes place. It requires a sender and receiver who both have their own ways of telling and hearing stories. In that sense communication is not only a message but also an act and interaction.

Virginia Satir (1972) was another therapist with lots to say about communication patterns in families. One of the many useful ideas was the idea of congruent and incongruent communication. She identified four major types of incongruent communication. The *Placator* is always nice to others but fails to say what they really feel – 'Whatever you want is OK'. The *Blamer* finds fault and dictates, and fails to acknowledge the other's perspective – 'You never do anything right'. The *Computer* (super-rational) is reasonable and logical but fails to acknowledge their own emotions – If one were to observe carefully. And finally, the *Distractor* often goes on about irrelevant matters in a ditzy way but is not really present at all – 'Burble, ho ho, burble!'

By contrast, the congruent communicator is aware of self and of his or her own feelings, aware of the other and their thoughts and feelings and aware of the surroundings and appropriateness of different levels of communication.

- Sharing the illness story
- Reducing the pace
- Normalising the impact of the illness
- Examining and re-framing illness narratives
- Addressing communication difficulties
- Addressing losses and gains
- Preparing for the future.

Next please . . .

Jade C was, yet again, an extra on the morning surgery. Her mother, a single woman with four children, came in looking apologetic and frazzled all at the same time. Jade, now two and a half and completely at home in the consulting room, had been burning up and coughing. Both mother and the health visitor knew that Mrs C had had a terrible experience three years ago when her baby had died of meningitis. No one had been to blame but she had found it difficult to regain any sense of confidence in her ability to judge illness in her children since. This time the health visitor decided to take an extra few minutes: 'I know how difficult it is for you to feel confident since you lost Abie three years ago. Is there anything, or anyone you feel would help you regain some confidence?' Mrs C appeared quite unsure for a while. The health visitor looked at the family tree and showed it her: 'Is there anyone on here who could help you regain your confidence?' 'Well, my grandmother could have done, but she died last year.' The HV had not known that. They talked about what it was about the grandmother that would have helped: 'If she was here, how do you think she might have helped you?' These speculations and another two sessions where the HV went over the Baby Check tool all helped a little. The children grew up and Mrs C, although still on the anxious side, was less often around the practice.

Next please . . .

Mr E, age 48, had been diagnosed with cancer of the lung a while ago. Over the past two years he had survived chemotherapy and surgery. It was after yet another chest infection and some weight loss, some six months ago, that his 14-year-old son John developed a chronic cough. No medication seemed to cure it and the GP was convinced that it was a 'nervous cough'.

Giving this 'diagnosis' to John did not help. John and both his parents asked for his care to be transferred to another 'more sympathetic' doctor, Dr S, in the health centre. Dr S requested for the whole family to attend 'so that I get a full picture about what everyone thinks about this cough'. Both parents came and so did John and his 5-year-old sister Betty. Dr S enquired what each family member thought about the causes of John's persistent cough. Mr E talked about a 'prolonged cold that's got stuck in John's throat'. John's mother remarked that 'coughs run in the family'. Betty said she thought that it was because John was smoking secretly 'just like dad'. Mr E looked alarmed and denied that he had been smoking during the past two years. It was then John's turn and, bursting into tears, he said: 'Dad . . . I see you smoking, up the chimney, when nobody is looking.' It was precisely at this point that Mr E broke into a major coughing fit. Once he had stopped, Mrs E turned to her husband and asked: 'Is that true?' Mr E sheepishly admitted it. Everybody looked at the floor. There was a deadly silence. Suddenly John started coughing. Mrs E said: 'I think you are coughing because nobody dares to talk about dad's cough.' It then emerged that the family had never talked together about Mr E's cancer. Dr S met with the family on three further occasions, for double appointments. Slowly, everybody talked about their hopes and fears, making preparations for the future. Mr E stopped smoking and John's cough stopped at the same time.

C – Community resources

Patients and their families do not live in some kind of vacuum – even though some clinicians treat them as if they did. We live in neighbourhoods, with corner shops and community centres. We visit temples, synagogues, mosques or churches. Our social support network includes friends, schools, youth clubs and other settings. Members of the primary care team usually have good knowledge of local resources, whether mother and toddler groups, or the local Newpin or Surestart initiatives. There may be family centres, lunch-time clubs for the elderly or groups for people with special issues. Clinicians who think 'systems' may well prefer these resources to medication or formal counselling.

It is also helpful to find out from patients what they regard as their local resources, and the Family Circles Method (Chapter 6) lends itself well to such an exploration:

> *I would like to find out with you what supports you have in your life, whether friends, neighbours, extended family, shopkeepers, local clubs – or whatever. Why don't you think about these for a few minutes and put them in this circle?*

There are times when knowing about the available and accessible community resources can be very helpful. An acute episode of illness can require intensive care at home or hospitalisation. The family's support network will determine to what extent the patient can be managed in the home environment. Here family and friends may play an important role and the clinician needs to evaluate the family's social ties and support systems.

E – Environmental factors

It must be obvious that the environment within which patient and family live is an important factor for their health. We know that poverty, bad nutrition and poor housing are all significant risk factors for people's physical and emotional health. For patients with physical disabilities environmental modifications are often crucial for improving the quality of their lives. Primary care clinicians get directly involved

Entering the political arena

Randomly select three patients you have seen in a day. Ask yourself the following questions:

- What do I know about the patient's actual living conditions?
- What is the financial situation for this family – and how is each person affected by it?
- How is the living environment adapted to the patient's disability?
- If I was this patient's MP, what might I want to fight for on their behalf?
- If there was one social or political change I could make to improve the patient's health, what might that be?

Discuss your findings with a radical friend!

in the practicalities of certain issues and find themselves writing letters to housing departments and benefit agencies. Yet, 'thinking families' means also 'thinking larger systems', such as considering how the larger social, cultural and political context is affecting the health of the family. Stopping short of intervening here can mean that one inadvertently confirms the 'pathology' of the family, rather than examining how society's pathologies contribute to the family's suffering. But then, where do the responsibilities of primary care clinicians end? Each reader may need to find their own answer to how political clinicians can and should be.

Assessing our patients along various different dimensions can produce many new ideas, not just for us as clinicians but, more importantly, for our patients and their families. But sometimes, before acting on some of these ideas, it is useful to find some time for reflection, the moment when you privilege thinking over doing. There is opportunity for more systemic work before or after the patient is seen. The 10 minutes we give our patients – or the 20 minutes we reserve for double appointments – often do not allow any 'time out' for systemic reflection. When faced with a patient's intense request and feeling under a lot of pressure to 'deliver', the clinician's creative thinking can get blocked and old consultation practices will resurface.

From assessing to reflecting – beyond the looking glass

So, you have been doing a lot of reading in the first half of the book – and now it is time to reflect. Here is a framework for systemic reflection. Reflection is probably the most important and least valued activity in primary care settings. It is a reactive world. If there are patients to be seen, then out with the break, out with

Time to spare

Time is the biggest issue for many people working in primary care. It organises much of our thinking and behaviour. It is often invoked as a reason for not being able to consult differently. In the last chapter we will look at barriers to change in the consultation, but for now it may be worth reflecting on some of the evidence about consultation length.

There is now good evidence that the length of consultation can be used as a proxy for quality and that usually it directly correlates with the number of problems, issues or topics identified and addressed (Howe 1996).

It is our belief that investing adequate time, particularly towards the 'front end' of problems, when they are newer and have not been practised and ingrained for so long, pays dividends. Identifying and addressing somatisation early on will save the patient, their family, you and the system much money and grief. The same is often true in those 'strange loop' consultations when you end up feeling that you and the patient did not find a meeting, a shared understanding of what was going on. It pays to spend the time working it out before six more fruitless consultations have gone by.

There is a wealth of literature on how to use time better, but we recommend you start by discussing with other practitioners who have found time to reflect – just how they manage it.

the coffee time, out with lunch – let's see the patients. But without reflection it is doubtful we can learn. So we need to make time for it.

In previous chapters we have sung the praises of an ever-curious and questioning approach. We have described how our patients get 'infected' by this and how a mutual search for new solutions can begin, involving both patient and clinician. We have described various techniques on how to build up, bit by bit, a picture of the patient and the (usually invisible) family. These include the use of genograms in one consultation and family circles in another. Over time more new information emerges, the clinician is able to move from having hunches to forming hypotheses. In the light of feedback and further information, new hypotheses are evolved and old ones discarded. Sharing one's ideas with patients involves them in the assembly of what could be seen as a giant jigsaw puzzle.

The making of hypotheses and the attempts to corroborate them is an important activity in physical and psychological medicine and in other areas of scientific enquiry. It is also important in primary care. It aids the diagnostic process and the formulation of a treatment or management plan. However, all too often the patient is excluded from being actively involved in this process. Of course, it is possible to come up with ideas, even if they are 'wild' or 'informed', *before* the consultation with a patient. The clinician will be organised by questions such as: 'Why has he made another appointment for today – I only saw him yesterday?' or 'I saw granny two days ago, her daughter yesterday and now they're bringing the grandchild with some minor problem – what on earth is going on in this family?' The clinician can attempt to answer these questions speculatively, knowing that any emerging hypotheses are not 'truths'. They are working tools that focus the enquiry, that need to be tested and that have to be modified – or thrown out altogether – in the light of the information that emerges. New hypotheses can then be put forward and guide further enquiry.

We have, in fact, already done lots of work on hypothesising in the previous chapters, encouraging you to use the different perspectives generated to explore different hypotheses. What we want to do now is expand and add complexity to your hypothesis making! Go on, we think you are ready for it. We want to look in more detail at culture, race and gender.

Extending hypothesising

Consider the following case example which could be examined from a whole variety of different angles, based on the PPRACTICE model, thus generating many, too many, hypotheses. Here we will just concentrate on a few dimensions.

Next please . . .

Ms D is a 45-year-old woman from Jamaica. She has lived in England for some 20 years. She has four children, from three different fathers – ranging from 2 to 24 years of age. Her oldest, Jenny, was mostly brought up by Ms D's own mother. Jenny is now a single parent herself and has two children of her own. Ms D's two teenage children, Billy and Ella, grew up with her second partner who died suddenly four years ago. Both are at present going through a lively adolescence. Their mother has indicated that she wants to return permanently to Jamaica, as the father of the youngest child, Jo, lives there. Ms D, Jenny, Billy and Ella are all multiple attenders, presenting mostly with psychosomatic complaints. There has recently been a spate of appointments with several members of the family. The clinician is struggling to cope and it is clear that Billy is unhappy at the moment.

A brief glance at the practice model would reveal the following two-minute overall assessment:

- *Problem*: Billy unhappy, doctor stuck.
- *Problem solving*: identified a problem but not discussed nor brainstormed within the family. GP awaiting case discussion.
- *Affect*: close family able to express some distress.
- *Time in the life cycle*: significant bereavement and adolescent children facing a possible move.
- *Illness*: somatising their distress.
- *Community/culture*: Jamaican family in England.
- *Environment*: possible issues of poverty and racism.

The clinician concludes that out of these areas it would seem most profitable to tackle the time in the life cycle issues and the issues to do with culture, race and community. Help in these areas would meet the family's and doctor's needs to get unstuck.

All of us are full of conscious or unconscious cultural, sexist, racist and classist beliefs and practices. All of us? Surely not you, dear reader! Well that's why we are asking you to address yourself to the questions asked in these two boxes. It has been argued by a variety of authors (McGoldrick 1998) that our discriminatory beliefs and practices not only define what gets labelled as a 'problem', but also the responses society puts in place.

Culture and gender 1

- Speculate on what the issues might be in this family.
- Consider how your own race, culture, gender, life experience and social context may have influenced your thoughts in relation to this family.
- What prejudices might you have?
- What do you know about Afro-Caribbean culture?
- Is it just one culture or do we conveniently, and stereotypically, lump together many diverse cultures under the same umbrella?
- Is this family's constellation 'typical' within this context – or is it 'abnormal'?
- What does it say about the role of women and the position of men in that culture?
- What do you know about culture-specific child-rearing patterns?
- How do individuals from different cultures somatise psychological issues?
- How do their expectations of medical services differ?
- How might they respond to our questions which are perhaps based on different expectations of normality?
- How do you manage when you are presented with a family about whose culture you feel you know very little?

Culture and gender 2

- How can curiosity about the cultural dimension help you to understand this family's symptoms and behaviours?
- How is a Jamaican family living in England for 20 years different from a white English family living in England?
- How is a white English family living in Jamaica different from a black Jamaican family living in Jamaica?
- If some of the fathers of Ms D's children had been white British, how might that dimension have been incorporated into the family's new story?
- How are your professional responses organised by cultural and other contextual presentations?

Making contextual hypotheses and formulating interventions – some further ideas

This section concerns itself with reflective practice: sometimes thinking about the more complex issues – even though it may well take 10 minutes! – saves time in the long run. To arrive at more comprehensive ideas, there are a number of questions clinicians can pose for themselves, to guide their exploration.

What is the family configuration and life cycle stage? Which relationships are entering or undergoing a transition?

In Ms D's family we have children of three different ages and life cycle transitions: one who has left home, two who are engaged in adolescent behaviours and a charming toddler. This information permits the making of a series of different hypotheses.

- *Hypothesis 1*: The death of the teenagers' father was an important family life cycle event which presented Ms D with the responsibilities of being a single parent.
- *Hypothesis 2*: The arrival of a new man and baby has created an imbalance in the family. There is concern in the family that he will pull them apart, this cannot be discussed and is therefore presented via physical symptoms.
- *Hypothesis 3*: The family is having to cope with adolescence at a time when it still mourns the loss of paternal father. This might have the effect of putting off home-leaving, at least for the time being.
- *Hypothesis 4*: The family structure is a usual Jamaican family responding to bereavement by the leaving home of other family members. They regard themselves as 'normal'.

Enshrined in these hypotheses, which are different and at the same time complementary, are beliefs about adolescence that are mediated by culture. For example, in most North American and North European contexts, individualism and individuality are important concepts by which people live and structure lives. Individual decision making, personal self-esteem and self-worth, personal responsibility, individual human rights are all expressions of a strong belief in the 'self' – and this notion very much affects the goals clinicians have for bringing about change in the patients and families they see.

Therapeutic endeavours traditionally aim to strengthen the 'self', helping the person to 'individuate'. Such interventions may be quite misplaced with patients who come from communal, collectivistic or extended family cultures, where questions relating to the 'self' are often experienced as intrusive, insensitive and rude (Waldegrave 1998). For example, a Samoan, when asked a question like 'What do you think about this . . . ?' will find it difficult to answer directly. Instead he or she may reflect: 'What does my mother think? What does my grandmother think? What does my father think? What does my uncle think? What does my brother think? What is the consensus of those thoughts? Yes, that must be what I think' (Waldegrave 1998).

When asking questions in a family context, issues of intergenerational respect may be very prominent in specific cultures and affect the meanings attributed to these very questions. Ms D said that she was brought up by her parents and grandparents to have utter respect for them and not to challenge their views. The clinician interviewing her may start by asking her about her views regarding her teenage children's behaviour and, once having elicited these, turn to Billy and Ella and ask: 'You both have heard what your mum said about you. What are your views about what she thinks about your behaviour?'

Being asked to comment on the observations of the parental generation individualises the teenager. This may go against cultural conventions. Moreover, encouraging teenagers to voice their opinions and differences may be experienced by the parent or elders as disrespect. Clinicians who are unfamiliar with or insensitive to such cultural mores will inadvertently break cultural taboos and be at risk of setting up a confrontation between two generations.

How do the presenting problems reflect cultural patterns?

In individualistic cultures healthy development is usually equated with leaving home and differentiation and individuation from the family of origin, permitting the formation of 'outside' relationships with a partner. Clinicians employing this framework tend to view lifelong inter-dependence and connectedness with one's parents as 'problematic'. Yet, there are plenty of societies and social minorities whose life conditions and economic realities make the parent–child relationship more important and stable than the partnership or the marital bond (Falicov 1998). For example, the 'familial self' of Japanese and Indians contrasts strongly with the 'individual self' of mainstream Americans. Here the enduring emotional connectedness and involvement with the family of origin is a key value. Maintaining both the reputation and honour of the family of origin seems more important than nurturing and maintaining relationships with 'outsiders'. Furthermore, in many collectivistic extended families, leadership and authority tend to be located in the older generation, often with patriarchal privileges, with men having public authority over women (Falicov

1998). Yet, there are also distinct matriarchal families, with men seemingly relegated to the mere role of sperm donors.

It has been observed that the messages given to black African American men and women about gender roles and expectations are often contradictory and confusing (Boyd-Franklin and Franklin 1998). One message for black women is not to be dependent on black men, as they cannot be trusted to stay with and provide for women and children. Another simultaneous message given is that a woman's goal is to find a black man who will take care of her. The resulting bind often leads to complex relationship issues. Black men also are often given mixed messages by their families of origin: 'be assertive, productive and dominant . . . but don't be too aggressive, or too dominant, because the white man will cut you down'. Black males learn to be 'cool', often hiding any inner emotional turmoil behind a mask of total composure (Boyd-Franklin 1989, Majors and Billson 1992).

So how can clinicians cope with these complex issues with regard to culture, ethnicity and race? The clinician's position of 'informed not-knowing' is a useful one. It represents an aspiration to be as informed as possible about those we perceive as being different and, by implication, about ourselves and the beliefs and prejudices we hold. It is possible to gather this information from very different sources: books, journeys, friends, TV and radio and, most importantly, patients. We also need to be aware of the danger of cultural stereotypes and remember that there is a lot of within-group diversity. One can never assume common sets of meanings within any one grouping. In fact, being aware of the broader cultural context to which our patient belongs helps us to ask: 'How is *this* patient performing culture?' As informed not-knowers, from a position of 'safe uncertainty' (Mason 1993), we have to listen 'radically'.

So where does that leave our hypothesising with regard to Ms D's family? What were and are the belief systems about who cares for whom and for what periods of time? There are many challenges for the clinician working with Ms D, whether the

Family of origin (FOO) group work

'Know thyself' is a tall order and a life-long task. There are multiple tools that can help to gain some level of insight about oneself in relation to others, whether partners or patients. One of the ways we have found useful is to pull together a small group of colleagues into a FOO group. This is the systemic version of a Balint seminar group (Balint 1957, Salinsky and Sackin 2000). Balint's contribution was to make it clear that both the doctor and the patients are active subjects in the consulting room. The clinician is not neutral and objective, their own narratives, experiences and prejudices are present and open to transference and all the other psychological processes. What systemic perspectives do is to encourage further exploration of family of origin amongst the members of the group. To look at beliefs, cultural background, birth order and various other organising contexts that go to make up who we are, all these help us to understand how we behave. FOO groups work at the meeting place between patients, stories and the clinicians' own lives. It is fascinating how often an examination of the clinician's genogram in the context of talking about a specific worrying patient helps shed light on why the clinician is worried.

clinician is white middle class and born in Surrey or, like Ms D, born and bred in Jamaica and now navigating life in twenty-first-century England. One of the issues is of course that of somatising and frequent attendees. It will not be possible for all clinicians to become outstanding culturally informed practitioners or to know the details of multiple different cultures. But the diversity of patients seen in British primary care is growing all the time and so some culture-sensitive skills are required! Perhaps the most useful thing we can do is to adopt Shapiro's stance of 'not knowing'.

The following phrases are often useful:

- 'You know Ms D, can you be my teacher on this one? How far do you feel the kids are influenced by your origins in Jamaica and how much by their lives here in the UK? In my experience many young people get symptoms in their bodies when their minds are unhappy or not relaxed. Do you have a similar idea?'
- 'If I had been Billy's doc in Jamaica, what might you have imagined me to say about Billy's current behaviour?'
- 'Is it OK for me to ask Billy what his thoughts are?'
- 'If your mother had been sitting with us what would she have said about Billy's behaviour?'

How does the social situation affect the symptoms?

The social situation comprises a whole variety of contexts, from the neighbourhood to other settings and groupings which are defined by geography, work, religion or ethnicity. Experiences of being subjected to racism, social exclusion because of poverty or prejudice, all these are issues that could affect the well-being of any member of Ms D's family. For many black Afro-Caribbean families the church and congregation play a major role for identification, hope and support: enlisting the help of the preacher may well be the most appropriate and effective intervention.

What function does the symptom serve in stabilising the family? and How does the family (and each member) function in stabilising the symptom?

Ms D's family presents with more than just one problem: in fact, different members of the family present with a whole range of different psychosomatic symptoms. Perhaps that is the only way in which individuals in this family can communicate to each other about being distressed. Any talk about the loss of father, or the possible 'loss' of mother to the husband-in-waiting, is taboo. It revives too many painful feelings from the past and fears of abandonment in the future. The symptom, multiple presentations at the health centre, stabilises the family in that it keeps the family's Pandora box firmly shut. Yet, the price seems high, with each person having to be ill to stabilise the family.

Translating speculation into action

Pooling all these ideas is not only time consuming but can also be highly confusing: where does one start? Most clinicians do not have the time to sit back and brood over the many possibilities arising from the above questions. But then, perhaps we spend our time uneconomically. In our efforts to find solutions we are at pains to take complex histories, examining what need not be examined, prescribing what we know will not help and keeping our fingers crossed that some magic will happen before we have to see the patient again. Systemic therapists working in specialist settings with co-therapists, videos or one-way screens do take time out with colleagues to discuss families. These facilities are rarely available to family clinicians, but it is occasionally a very effective use of time to take five minutes before, during or after a consultation to think. Would patients be more or less satisfied if the clinician said the following?

> *This problem seems difficult to me and I need to think about it by myself for a few minutes. I would like to stop this consultation for, let's say, about five minutes so that I can have some time to reflect about some of the issues that have been raised and we can then reconvene.*

The clinician can leave the consulting room or ask the patient to go to the waiting area of the surgery or clinic. Taking 'time out' is often useful and, ironically, results in a shorter consultation.

In the next case, Mr and Mrs I have a problem (P) in that they are both ill. They have not really thought that they have a problem to solve (P). They are muddled in their roles (R) but actually care a great deal for each other (A). They appear to communicate (C) by Mr I being recurrently ill. They are at a transitional stage of retirement (T). Illness (I) is a major part of the picture. They have not accessed their community (C) nor family resources adequately. We know little about whether they are adequately housed and provided with benefits (E).

Next please . . .

Mr I is 60 and his wife is also 60. He has been off work since a neck injury 10 years ago. She has had a heart complaint for five years, so he has to do more around the house. They have four grown-up children who live nearby. Mr I does all the housework except for food preparation. He has stopped driving because of neck pain when turning the steering wheel. He also tends to work too hard in the home and then gets very bad pain. His appointments with physiotherapy were unsuccessful because the exercises did not make the pain go away. Discussing the pain Mr I says the advantage of working hard is that he does not notice the pain at the time, he gets things done and he feels a certain sense of pride. He says something is missing in his life since he stopped work. All the housework boosts his self-esteem. Mrs I praises him, as do other members of the family. Mr I says the disadvantages are that he does not sleep well for worrying about how it will all get done, as well as panicking about the future. He gets exhausted every few days, becoming irritable and his wife is cross with him, feeling unfit herself and becoming generally demoralised. During the consultation with Mr I it emerged that one of the blocks preventing him from pacing himself effectively had to do with his beliefs about how men have to provide for the family. He talked about being a perfectionist ('I come from a family of perfectionists'), believing that no one, especially not his children, could do the jobs well enough. Mr I also thought that his wife was locked into thinking that she would get worse if she stretched herself and so she indirectly encouraged his behaviour.

The GP challenged both when he saw them in the next consultation, by asking these questions:

- *'Supposing you took it in turns to take each other tea in bed in the morning, what would that be like for you both?'*
- *'What would be the advantages and disadvantages?'*
- *'Supposing you did this as an experiment for two weeks starting from tomorrow, how would you decide who got tea in the morning?'*
- *'Supposing you both wanted to test out how helpful your children could be in an emergency and decided to be uncharacteristically mischievous and Mr I took to his bed for three days saying he was ill when he was not. Which of your children would respond first? Which second? Which last?'*
- *'Supposing you decided that the children needed to cook Sunday lunch for you both once a month, who would you ask first? What would be the benefits and difficulties of doing this?'*
- *'Supposing I referred you to the physiotherapist again but with a clear message that she was to give you gentle exercises to improve your general physical fitness so that you could cope better with more stamina. I don't think she can do anything much for the day-to-day pain. Would that be acceptable?'*
- *'Supposing you planned your week carefully to pace all that needs to be done (shopping, cooking, housework, etc.) what would you do? How would that be different from how you organise your week now?'*
- *'Supposing you changed some of these things we have talked about, who would feel most anxious? What usually happens to such anxiety? How long does it take to settle?'*

Mr and Mrs I smiled quite a bit in this consultation, faced with these hypothetical questions and struggling with possible answers. Six weeks later they reported that 'we are now job sharers'. They had worked out the roles in their lives differently.

 Time out for clinicians

The next time you find yourself in a very difficult consultation:

- Tell the patient that you need a 'five-minute break to think about the complex issues raised, just by myself'.
- Send the patient to the waiting room.
- Pretend that you are an outside observer who has just witnessed the consultation between yourself and the patient.
- Imagine what this observer might say, first positive and then negative comments.
- Imagine what a systemic clinician might do (look at one of the Fruits boxes you have copied out of this book if you are stuck!).
- Once the patient has returned, note the effect of your time out on the rest of the consultation.
- Tell the patient that you are stuck – if you are – and ask the patient to help you to come up with some novel ideas.

Practice makes perfect!

Having access to a CD-ROM hypothesiser that could sit in your head would be a great piece of computer software. Keeping the framework of PPRACTICE in your head and adding circular questions to them to elicit further ideas is the next best thing – it also reminds you of areas often forgotten about like underlying feelings and the income status of our patients. Practice makes perfect!

P = Problem
P = Problem solving
R = Roles
A = Affect
C = Communication
T = Time in life cycle
I = Illness experience
C = Community
E = Environment

Working with couples   9

This chapter covers:
- ○ Practical issues when working with more than one person
- ○ Indications for couple work
- ○ Convening the couple
- ○ Externalising the relationship
- ○ Dealing with domestic violence

Frequently, in consultations, primary care clinicians find themselves sitting with more than one potential patient. We have already described how it is possible to do couple and family work by invoking the virtual presence of other family members by way of questioning and pondering with the family member who is present. There may be times when you welcome having someone else in the room, who, although apparently just coming 'for support', may help to 'shift' or change the consultation. You may just be fascinated to discover that two people you have seen independently are in fact related or you may find yourself intrigued that the person you have been consulting with for years actually *has* a partner! You ask yourself: 'How did he fade out of the conversations I have had with her all this time?' On the other hand, what do you do if a female patient insists on bringing her husband? What if an adult patient turns up with his mother? What if a couple decide, without any warning, to come together, so that you can deal with their marital problems? Or perhaps you decide that the only way forward is to invite both partners along? Then who is your patient? How do you start? How do you manage confidentiality issues? How do you set about working with a couple? It may feel that having more than one person in the room is the last thing you want.

This chapter addresses both the practical issues and the many indications and rewards of seeing couples in primary care settings whether you felt you wanted them there or not! Most of these couples will tend to be partners, but on occasions adult 'child'/parent couples may present with very similar dynamics. On the whole in this chapter we are talking about adult/adult pairs rather than adult and child. Some may worry that we are offering primary care clinicians a quick course in how to do couple therapy. It is our belief that there is no rigid distinction between therapy and 'not therapy'. It is a continuum of skills. All that we offer here are some thoughts on how to increase the therapeutic effectiveness of clinicians in primary care settings and this is why we are talking about couple work rather than therapy.

Therapy or consultation?

This idea of therapy as distinct from consultation is an interesting one. It seems to us that the very idea of deciding to come (or, in some cases, not to come) to see a clinician may be therapeutic. Therapy comes from the Greek word for 'attendance' – a therapist is someone who attends to a patient. The solution-focused therapists pay great attention to what changes have already started to occur before the client even arrives, seeing these as worthwhile evidence of the strengths and ability to change that the patient brings themselves.

Within a simple 10-minute consultation major changes can occur. Every question is an intervention in bringing forth new thoughts and possible ways of thinking and feeling. It is like leaving a clean field before the patient as they enter the room and waiting for the opening gambit; this can be a challenge but a rewarding one (Neighbour 1987).

Starting the consultation with the words 'So, what are we doing today?' signals a collaborative mode of work and it may well elicit different and more useful possibilities to the more usual 'SO, what can I do for you?' which is a doctor-centred opening.

Just think about how we define therapy in a profession-centred way: it is something therapists do! Might it not free both ourselves and our patients to think that therapy is something that we all might do from time to time?

Indications for involving partner

Couple sessions in primary care can be initiated by the clinician or by one or both partners. Let us look at some of the situations when it might be appropriate for the clinician to consider inviting the partner to attend the next consultation in person.

- The patient hints repeatedly that he or she has a 'two-person problem' – defined as marital, sexual or behavioural.
- Frequent, separate ('parallel') attendances by different family members.
- Concordance problems when working with patients who have a chronic illness.
- Acute family crisis (sudden death, baby blues, parasuicide, drug misuse in family member).
- 'Heartsink' patients (O'Dowd 1988) and 'stuck' consultations.
- Depression in either partner.
- Health behaviours – smoking cessation, hypertension.

Advantages of working with couples

As you might have guessed, we believe there are many opportunities offered by having more than just one person in the consulting room. There is often an advantage from the patient's point of view too: surprisingly, many patients actually do like to have someone from their own life involved in consultations. It makes total sense to them, but they are often not asked. One small study (R. Bothelho, personal communication) found that at least 50 per cent of clients brought at least one other person into the waiting room. Very few brought them into the consultation but 50 per cent said they would have liked to bring that other person in if given 'permission' to do so.

Health centre poster

Not so long ago it was not uncommon (and probably still is in some places) to find signs in waiting rooms that say things like 'Please do not bring anyone else to the appointment with you' or 'Each appointment is for one person only – please make another appointment if you need one'. These are classic examples of doctor-, service- or professional-centred ideas.

Here is a form of words you can display on a poster in your health centre:

Seeing your doctor, nurse or health visitor?
Please feel free to bring a partner, spouse or friend to your
appointment if you feel it would be helpful for you

Traditionally, doctors and patients have usually thought it best to have just the two of them in the consulting room. However there are a number of times when it may be useful to bring someone with you:

- When you feel you need support, or someone to 'remember what the doctor or nurse said'.
- When someone else may help with understanding the problem or, more importantly, perhaps they may help with thinking about the solution.
- When the issue to be discussed is a joint one.
- When it just feels right.

Family and friends are often very important and useful and we are always happy to see them with you. Of course that doesn't mean we can solve all the family's problems in one 10-minute appointment! But it does sometimes help a lot with thinking about YOU.

Another person always widens the field of observation and provides another perspective on 'the problem', symptom or illness. Furthermore, clinicians can observe the partner interactions 'in vivo' and get a flavour of what the difficulties are. Have you ever noticed how differently some patients present when in the company of a relative compared with being seen on their own? Having seen both individuals, what you have heard makes you think that there is a 'his marriage' and a 'her marriage', because they seem to have described the 'same' relationship completely differently. Interventions can be designed that address the directly observed behaviours and communication styles there and then.

Some of the worries about three-person consultations

On many occasions we do not think three is a crowd. But you, and on some occasions your patients, may not feel it is a good idea. And this may be for good reasons. You may be concerned about time, about the skills you will need, or about confidentiality. Patients may share these and other concerns. They may feel that they have struck up a good and trusting relationship with their clinician and believe that bringing the partner might spoil this. Moreover, some patients may have confided things that their spouses do not know about, maybe discussing an affair or another 'secret' issue from the past. Confidentiality issues can be complex, raising considerable dilemmas: if one of the partners is the known patient, will the other partner perceive the clinician as biased? How might this impact on the interviewing style? If the clinician attempts to be 'neutral', will the patient feel let down? After all, the patient may have dragged the partner along – 'just so he can hear it from the doctor'! Which aspects of a patient's life, based on prior knowledge, can the clinician talk about and which not? How can the clinician know – or even remember – which of the information is meant to be 'classified' and which not? What if the clinician is placed in a position where it becomes apparent that the patient is lying to the partner – and the patient knows that the clinician knows? What if both partners consult the clinician frequently and each has shared privately secrets or other sensitive information? Here each partner knows that the clinician knows these particular secrets and probably both also suspect that the clinician knows a bit more than he or she lets on. Knowingly or unknowingly the clinician can get caught up in a complex 'couple war' and take a lot of 'flak'. Seeing couples in primary care brings some potential difficulties, and it is understandable that many clinicians shy away from the idea. But, as you will see, there are ways of managing the offer of 'holding a secret', and respecting confidences.

Clinicians also often believe, rightly or wrongly, that they do not have the skills to do couple work. Some clinicians are able to acknowledge this and then choose to acquire these skills. Others may feel that what is needed is referral to an expert couple therapist. Sadly, not much comes of many of these referrals as the formality of such a referral dramatises the couple issue, making it 'official', with patients often stating that 'things aren't that bad'. Sometimes clinicians are rightly concerned that asking the partner to come will make things worse subsequently, with punitive actions – even violence – following such couple consultations. It is important to bear this possibility in mind and look at or ask about it. There are times, very occasionally, when couple work should carry a Health Warning.

Clinicians may also fear that one of the negative outcomes could be that the partners separate subsequently. This is indeed possible – though rarer than you think. But, are clinicians really that powerful? Even if a clinician wanted to 'prescribe' a separation, there is no evidence that patients comply with such 'medical advice'. People generally make their own decisions even if there is a tendency to blame others for what has gone wrong. A breakup is not always a bad outcome for couples in distress. Many people have a 'terminal care' view of relationship breakdown rather than seeing it as having possibilities for a 'complete remission' of life's miseries. It can pay to be as up-front about this issue as you would be about other areas of people's lives and to challenge your own and the prevailing cultural assumptions. Clinicians can probe:

> *Supposing you both decided to make a really good job of separating – one that you could be proud of – how would you achieve it? What would your relationship look like in two years' time? How would your children be with it all?*

How could you enable a good outcome for them? How would you deal with your extended family to help them feel proud of what you had achieved? What would a successful management of your financial separation look like?

And when mentioning what feels to be the unmentionable, here are some further openings:

Just supposing, as a result of all these difficulties, you decided to separate. What would be the advantages and disadvantages for you both?

Sometimes the thought of real marital breakdown is so scary that it doesn't get talked about and it acts like a lead weight in the marriage. So, one of the things I find often helps couples to sort out their difficulties in the present is to take an imaginary look into the future and look at the problems now from the position of you both living apart. What do you think and feel about that hypothetical situation?

Working with more than one person, and particularly the partner of the patient, can be hugely rewarding and effective. When the above issues are addressed, they can be overcome, opening up new avenues to deal with seemingly intractable symptoms or problems that have grown in a couple context.

Next please ...

Mrs D has been feeling very low for months. Previous consultations have revealed how much her depression is tied up with the behaviour of her husband, a man she repeatedly described as a workaholic. Circular and reflexive questions have established how her depression affects him and how his responses do not help her getting less depressed. Her doctor believes it is important to involve Mr D in the next consultation. However, Mrs D believes that she won't be able to persuade him.

How to get the partner to join you

In this case story the doctor first needs to discuss with the patient how she might get her husband to attend the next consultation. Furthermore, the doctor will also need to entertain the hypothesis that Mrs D may be very reluctant to bring him. One way of exploring such dynamics is to pose a series of questions:

What might you say to your husband to get him to come? Tell me what words you would actually use? And if he said that, how might you reply? So, if you predict that he would give a negative answer, how could you ask him differently, so that it would be more difficult for him to say 'no'?

Clinicians can rehearse, via 'question and answer' mini role play, various forms of words and the likely responses – and how these could, in turn, be responded to. Such mini rehearsals not only have a pragmatic value, but they may at times also reveal the patient's own resistance, in this case to bringing her partner. Further exploration and reassurances may be required:

- 'What might be the major disadvantages of your partner coming here?'
- 'What would be the worst outcome?'
- 'What might be the advantages?'
- 'If you had to weigh the pros and cons of your partner coming here with you, which way would the scales tip?'
- 'Are you concerned that it might change your relationship with me (or him)?'

It is also important to check out about violence and risk.

- 'Is there any risk that discussing these things might lead to violence or your partner hurting you?'
- 'Do you and your partner ever come to blows when you are discussing or arguing?'

It is only with the agreement of the patient that a joint consultation with a couple has a chance of being a useful next step. It is that old idea of concordance again – telling people to bring someone else is rarely effective if they have not explored the risks and benefits a bit first. Patients need to examine their hopes and fears before being plunged into what could be a confrontational encounter. For some patients it is seemingly 'easier' to blame the partner in absentia. They may be worried about upsetting the status quo, fearing that a can of worms will be opened. Such fears need to be explored respectfully first. Sometimes the very act of exploring the pros and cons of 'getting the partner in' reveal perhaps to both patient and clinician what is in fact going on.

- 'Well actually nurse, I think we have come to the end of the line. I am not sure, if I am really honest, I do want my marriage to work.'
- 'Well I know I complain a lot about him not helping enough with my legs and pains, but just talking about asking him makes me think that perhaps I have been ignoring his needs in all this. I think I need to talk about it with him first.'

But remember, if clinicians themselves do not feel convinced that it is important to have the partner in person in the consulting room, then this doubt will almost certainly be picked up by the patient. Clinicians' beliefs – and fears – clearly transmit themselves to their patients, who cannot help but respond in some way to these (often unspoken) communications. So have faith and try it out!

Turning an individual complaint into a couple issue

What is the potential counselling pathway for this woman? Talking as an individual would certainly help her to cope but would do little to address some of the likely issues between her and her husband. It would certainly not address any issues that he may have about having to be a good provider, being a success, worrying about his wife. The task, therefore, in the brief consultation is to explore whether her difficulty is more usefully seen in the context of her relationships, rather than within her as an individual needing to 'be made stronger': should her 'depression' be constructed and treated intra-personally or inter-personally? Here are some thoughts and questions that can guide this discussion.

- 'If your husband had listened to this conversation how would he be responding just now?'
- 'If we saw this problem as not belonging inside you but between the two of you, how would that help you decide what should happen next?'
- 'Supposing you have a role in your relationship to be a thermostat for family tensions, what is the best way for you to communicate your worries to your partner?'
- 'Does your partner understand your role as thermostat? If he did, how might he behave differently?'

Next please . . .

Mrs P is 36 and consulted feeling tired and irritable. She thinks she can't cope with her family and especially not her two teenage children. She has moved six times in the last six years, always following her husband's job. Recently she had got back pain and life had seemed even more unbearable. She had had a difficult relationship with her father but felt that she had grown through all that, unlike her sister, who was having counselling. Mrs P has no real friends because they have moved so much and last time she had also had to give up a job she really liked. She was beginning to feel resentful. She had come to the surgery wanting yet another 'magic' antidepressant, as well as counselling to make her stronger to cope with it all. The nurse's sense was that she seemed to be trying to cope with way too many things.

Same one, please . . .

Mrs P decided to go to see the practice counsellor who works with individuals and couples. In order to prepare her for the sessions, a discussion was opened up to help her think about how she might use the first one.

- *'If you went to the session on your own first, would it be more or less easy for your husband to attend next time?'*
- *'If you went together to the first session how easy would it be for you both to express most of what you wanted to say?'*
- *'If it would be difficult to say some important things, how could you let the counsellor know? How would it be if you asked your husband if you could both have some separate time before the session or even during the session?'*

Consulting to the partners

Let us assume that you and the index patient have managed to get the partner into the room. What now? When working with couples in short consultations it is important to have some basic rules in your mind:

- Anyone can leave the room.
- It is acceptable to ask the couple to stop arguing in front of you.
- It is very important to get a balanced idea of both partners' story/perspective on the problem.

Next please . . .

The practice nurse knew she had a double appointment with Mrs N, whose marriage was in difficulties. She had known her for many years as both her daughters were badly asthmatic. Mrs N phoned up 30 minutes before the appointment to say she was bringing her husband along as well. He wasn't a patient of the practice. The nurse voiced her concern that she knew Mrs N but not her husband so he might feel at a disadvantage, but said she was happy to see them both. The nurse opened the session by saying that they had 20 minutes and that to make best use of the time she would like to create a few ground rules: that it was important for everyone to have an opportunity to say what they wanted to say – and for the others to listen respectfully. She then added that if anyone of the three of them wanted some time out, they could leave the room to think more clearly. It was not long before Mr N blurted out that he was having an affair and mayhem ensued. Mrs N had suspected this and accused him of being 'a cheat and a liar'. He argued back as best he could. After two minutes of witnessing this, the nurse asked if the row was a helpful use of the time. Both paused and agreed that it was not. The nurse said she would like Mrs N to be just in a listening position for two minutes, so that she could get to know Mr N's view of the marriage and his reasons for having an affair. She indicated that she would ask Mrs N to comment on what her husband had said immediately afterwards.

* Mr N explained how he had never felt that they were 'a proper couple' because Mrs N was always around at her mum's and that he felt left out. He believed that all his hard work earning money was not appreciated. He then burst into tears and left the room. He returned after five minutes and they then spent some 10 minutes sharing the time to talk about some of the difficulties they had. The nurse summed up by congratulating them both on being able to attend together, reflecting that there was clearly plenty of discussion required for them to work out what future their relationship had. She offered to see them again to help them decide what way forward they would like. Afterwards she reflected briefly that, although she had not solved anything with or for them, she had successfully connected with the husband, as well as enabling the couple to have a constructive conversation, offering them the beginnings of a plan for working on their problems.*

Orienting couple work

When working with couples it is important to orient the consultation at the very outset. Here are a few suggested openings:

Thanks for coming here. You probably know that your partner has consulted me a number of times to do with the illness and symptoms. I suggested that it might be useful to meet with both of you together to see whether this could throw some light on the situation.

We do know that if one person is affected by depression that it can affect the partner – and the partner's responses and reactions in turn affect the person who is depressed. This is why I often like to invite those 'near and dear' so that I can see the larger picture.

Let me be quite clear that I did NOT ask you to come here today because I think that it is your fault that your partner is feeling low. I am just interested in your views about her illness/problem.

All this may seem long-winded or perhaps even over-cautious. However, it is our view that if considerable care is taken in orienting at the beginning, the consultation goes better. The first aim is to widen the perspective, to introduce some new ways of thinking about the symptomatic person and to involve the partner in this exploration, in the hope that this might affect the symptoms. Often clinicians do not have permission to make the relationship 'the problem'. The partner must not feel blamed and even if it is evident to the clinician that there is a 'relationship problem', it is unwise to challenge the partner's own way of seeing things at an early stage. Clearly this is different for partners who have both actively elected to bring their partnership issues for consultation.

However, in most situations we deal only with one 'identified' patient and clinicians often go out of their way to stress this, by confirming the established roles – namely one being the patient, the other being the 'suffering' partner. It is only when a couple are ready and give explicit permission to tackle relationship issues that clinicians should start working with these. Until that time clinicians are most successful if they respectfully treat the attending partner as someone who can provide valuable information about the patient's symptoms, problems or illness. It is through a gradual process of asking circular and reflexive questions that over time the tapestry of an interactional picture can be weaved:

- 'And when he is depressed, how does that affect you and other members of the family? How do you respond?'
- 'What do you think he finds most and least helpful?'
- 'If you wanted to make him feel more depressed – not that you would! – what might you have to do?'

Joining with each person and clarifying the issue

The initial stages of such work could best be described as joining with each partner and finding ways of engaging with both.

A safe way of starting may be to construct a joint family tree or genogram (see Chapter 5). This is particularly useful if you are actually meeting a newly registered couple for the first time (in fact this is often a great opportunity to try out a few of the ideas in this chapter). Try to make sure that both partners can see the family tree as you construct it. Look carefully for any non-verbal and other clues that new information has appeared that one partner did not know or register before: 'I told you that my uncle committed suicide – least I am sure I did – well I meant to certainly.' Non-verbal clues can be as subtle as a frown from one partner when the other describes the disciplinarian father she had. 'I come from a family of six and we had three different fathers, George is an only child – I sometimes think that must make a huge difference.'

Whether in the context of a genogram or simply in the process of engagement, even-handed attention needs to be given to each partner and to their beliefs, as well as their hopes and fears. Thus, even if these views are contradictory, by giving equal weight to each the clinician will, at one and the same time, communicate a desire to understand each partner, *and* will begin to offer the therapeutic suggestion that more than one point of view may be valid. This stance of even-handedness, and the sense of 'being in tune', can be communicated via words (e.g. reflecting

Blame and responsibility

The notions of blame and of responsibility have had an interesting time in the family therapy field. In the early days (see Chapter 3) it appeared that therapists were almost blaming the family for the illness of the identified patient. R.D. Laing's work might have been seen as advocating this position (Laing and Esterson 1964). It was certainly the way some families felt in therapy. Later ideas have moved far from this position. Indeed you could be forgiven for wondering whether the postmodern clinicians who believe the only reality is constructed in language actually believe anyone does anything 'wrong'. However, this newer and allegedly more 'modern' thinking has encouraged clinicians to be much more interested in how couples construct together the problems that they have. Each may bring particular behaviours, but the outcomes are in part dependent on the partnership.

Attribution of blame is very rarely helpful for you as a therapist. It has the tendency to solidify the problem dynamics. But the habit of blaming still permeates current thinking. The following can be a useful phrase: 'I rarely find it helpful to attribute blame. Let's just see what both of your opinions are and then see where we go from there.'

The *seed* for you to grow from this is:

Ask yourself the last time you were listening to one partner and buying into their idea that the whole problem was the fault of the partner whose wicked deeds were being described. It often happens in situations of domestic violence or alcohol misuse. Now this is tricky, because of course some people's behaviour *is* quite unacceptable and that person needs to take responsibility for it. However, you are not there to take sides, because it is highly likely that in taking sides you are simply mirroring what all that person's supporters have already said. So, fine to agree that certain behaviours are unacceptable, but *then* you are in the business of seeing what new steps the person in front of you can take.

language used by the couple themselves), conscious posture (e.g. mirroring) and tone (Jones and Asen 2000).

It is important to check continuously whether you have understood what each person is saying (e.g. 'Let me just check with you that I've got this right'). Thus

Joining

Joining is a crucial first step when working with couples – and individuals. It is the process of accommodation between clinician and couple, the search for some kind of 'fit' that will be good enough to allow explorations in a context of safety (Minuchin 1974). It is also often referred to as forming a therapeutic alliance and developing rapport. This type of joining is an ongoing process which needs to be maintained throughout the clinical work. It aims both to establish engagement *and* to facilitate change.

repetition, in slightly changed language, offers confirmation of being understood, emphasising what has been said. The clinician attempts to maintain a stance of neutrality towards ideas and thus does not directly challenge statements made by one or the other partner – even if they appear to be critical or negative. Sympathetic, non-judgemental listening is perhaps the key technique of engagement, signalling respect for how couples, despite what appear to be their best efforts, have become stuck in difficult relationship patterns. Premature challenging of their stuckness or early reframing of the partner as 'part of the problem' needs to be avoided for a couple of reasons at least. First, it is likely that the partner will not return for another consultation. Furthermore, it is very unlikely to be that simple, and one partner will often have already tried blaming the other – stepping into one partner's 'steps in the dance' is unlikely to help! When the partner is not well known and the patient is one of your 'regulars', it is often worth paying even more attention to the views of the partner. Relationships with regulars are rarely jeopardised by this and it conveys the message that you are keen to hear the views of the previously silent partner.

When interviewed respectfully, most partners will see themselves as the providers of some seemingly 'objective' information. The systemic clinician, however, will be mindful that this is just one version of events, the partner's narrative which is both separate and interwoven with others. Some relatives engage in long narratives about the patient's problems (or, perhaps more accurately, *their* problems with the patient!). The clinician will need to tolerate this for a while and may then broaden the discussion, by repeatedly soliciting the views of the index patient:

> PARTNER: 'And she gets very depressed and irritable and nobody can then get on with her . . . it is just dreadful . . . she is so low . . .'

> CLINICIAN: 'Mrs S, would you like to respond to what your husband has just said? Do you see it that way too? Do you agree with him that this is what happens? What is your explanation as to why he sees it that way?'

This intervention can prove to be useful, encouraging the patient to respond to what her partner has said, either agreeing or disagreeing. Looking for different views, including disagreements, and reflecting on the reasons for these together with each partner, can encourage the couple to examine issues together. Addressing rather than denying differences is a first step towards learning to resolve conflicts.

Externalising the relationship

When there are clearly identified couple issues, there are three patients in the room: both individuals and the relationship itself. This perhaps explains why the room seems so crowded when couples bring in a marital problem! This notion is helpful in many ways, not the least because it can begin to shift the blame away from individuals. It can be helpful to leave a chair for the marriage/relationship to sit in or use an object – an ornament or stone, perhaps, to represent the relationship, as it gives the problem more of a physical quality and allows for some interesting conversations. Here are questions that can sometimes allow both partners to look more dispassionately at their relationship as something for which they are jointly responsible:

- 'If the relationship could speak, what would it say needed to be happening to sustain it?' (This is great for stopping blaming in its tracks – We are talking about the life of the relationship not the behaviour of the partner now.)
- 'What hopes and fears have you both had for the relationship?'
- 'Describe how you get on with this thing called your marriage/relationship?'
- 'How would your children describe your relationship separate from seeing you as parents?'
- 'What hopes and fears do they have for your relationship?'

A chronic illness can often occupy the position taken by the relationship (see Chapters 10 and 11). This leads to enormous distress as the couple grieve the advent of the illness and the loss of their relationship.

Next please ...

Mr G is a 65-year-old man whose wife has diabetes with additional complications of peripheral vascular disease. She has recently had vascular surgery to unblock her iliac vessels and has become quite depressed. When invited to put Her Diabetes in one chair and their Relationship in another, they were shocked to realise that they believed they had no relationship left: 'life is all illness'. Careful enquiry helped them think of small things they could begin to do to help them get some sense of a relationship back.

Supposing this was a routine technique for every couple with chronic illness, how might people's adaptation to their illness change?

Getting concrete

Much of this process of attempting to listen neutrally and understand each partner not only helps form a relationship but also helps to clarify the issues that are of most importance to the couple. It is helpful all the time to try to move the issue from the vague and all-encompassing to the specific and particular – from 'I don't think he loves me any more' to the 'When I get in from work I really wish that we could have 10 minutes to share what has happened in my day as well as listen to what has happened in his'.

There are several 'nodal points' in the day of a life of a couple which can be useful to focus on, although what the nodes are will vary hugely, depending on the particular circumstances of the couple:

- How they say hello and goodbye to each other
- How they organise meals
- How they plan and do something together
- How they decide on household chores or childcare.

Focusing on the processes around these simple interactions can help to clarify many issues and use time economically.

Next please ...

Mr J and his wife, both in their sixties, came to see their GP having read an article about Asperger's syndrome being a possible, increasingly 'popular' diagnosis in adults. Mr J was sure he had 'it' and they both wanted referral to a couple therapist who could understand the condition. He described a complete lack of awareness of the other's emotional states, which had driven his wife to distraction over the years. He had been an engineer and was very good at practical problem-solving but quite hopeless at emotional problem-solving. The GP asked them to put their relationship into the chair. She was taken aback when he didn't understand what she meant. When he finally cottoned on that his Asperger's syndrome was meant to metaphorically 'sit' next to him, he became slowly able to describe 'it' as a little version of himself that he knew all about and that wasn't a problem to him. His wife described 'it' as a 'massive tangle of barbed wire'. Mr J was shocked by this very different description and he decided that it was his task to help her untangle the wires and explain himself to her. She said that it would be helpful if he could learn to understand her. The GP commented that this understanding was what relationships were all about. If Mr J was interested, he showed he was already learning about emotional skills.

Enactment – seeing and making it happen in front of your eyes

Sometimes it can be useful to encourage a direct display of what happens outside the room. This sort of enactment can often be a shortcut to what is really at stake. It is similar to the experience of seeing people on evening house calls. Somehow the drama of the acute event often sharpens the issues. Here are a few forms of words that encourage direct couple interaction in front of the clinician, aimed at eliciting 'live samples' of typical interaction and communication patterns:

- 'Would you like to respond to what your husband has just said? And what is your response to what your wife has just said?'
- 'If you had to reply to what your wife just said, what would you say? And what is your response to that? Tell him! He's there, just tell him!'
- 'Can you both talk about that for a few minutes, because it seems important. Keep it going, this is between the two of you. Ignore me for a minute.'
- [When partner turns to clinician] 'Don't tell me, tell him/her, s/he needs to hear this!' or 'Just keep the conversation going, talk to each other about that.'

Getting a couple to talk to each other can in itself be very therapeutic and resolve problematic situations. As this takes place in front of a third person, the partners are more likely to be constructive and this is what the clinician can then build on. In this way the clinician acts as catalyst, making possible an interaction that would, in this form, not usually take place. At times it may come to a full-blown argument, an often potentially embarrassing experience for the clinician. One way of stopping such an argument is to state:

I can see you are both very angry with one another and it sounds as if you have a lot of practice having such rows. I don't mind you doing this on your own, if this is what you want to do. But whilst we three are together I would like you to stop arguing so that we can discuss how not to have such arguments – this is of course only if you both decide that it would be a good idea to stop these major arguments.

So, let us examine what it is that makes you have such rows: What is it that he has got to do or say to get you going? What is it that she has got to do or say to get you going? What is it that you would have to say or do to get him mad at you? What is it that you would have to say or do to get her mad at you?

Such interventive questioning has two purposes. It takes the heat out of the situation if this is required. In most primary care settings it may not be acceptable to have such 'therapeutic' arguments going on, as colleagues may feel unable to pursue their clinical or administrative work with a major row going on next door. From the couple's point of view, however, it can help each partner to pinpoint their own triggers as well as identifying what triggers the spouse. As a result, partners can come to a position where they begin to see their dual roles and positions: reacting to and provoking further arguments. They begin to take a step back and become 'observers' of the phenomenon that is their relationship in action.

The limits of couple work

Primary care clinicians are limited in the scope of couple work not only by location and skill, but also by time. Within the context of a 10- or 20-minute consultation, there is not time and space to get much detail on the complexities of relationships. This is, in many respects, an advantage rather than a constraint. The aim of couple work in primary care is *not* to solve people's relationship issues. Instead, the aim is to get the assistance of the partner in tackling the symptoms or illness by broadening the frame. The partner is directly involved in managing the person he or she lives with. Such involvement is often crucial to moving on. In practice, it helps to have a tight focus, just on one particular issue. The more concrete and describable the issue, the more successful the work. Discussing some vaguely termed 'communication difficulties' usually leads nowhere. By contrast, concrete issues such as money matters, contact with in-laws, responding to suicidal behaviour, managing an unruly teenage daughter and other domestic crises are all topics which permit concrete exploration. Furthermore, following this exploration, the partners can be asked to find views of resolving that particular issue and developing strategies for bringing about change. Working with couples in the context of primary care may be usefully seen as problem-solving work, with one of the major aims to keep the heat out of their interactions (Dallos and Draper 2000). Clinicians can elicit accounts from both partners of the difficulties *and* strengths that they perceive. Attempts can then be made to clarify and negotiate a shared new story and to work with them

 Evaluation

The next time you see more than one person in the surgery, encourage them to talk to one another about an issue they have brought up. Use phrases such as 'Can you talk to him about that now' and 'Would you like to respond to that?!' to get some 'live' interaction in the consulting room. Record your observations about the consultation afterwards and identify areas of your own competence in conducting couple consultations. Evaluate your own position *vis-à-vis* the couple and speculate about whose side each of them thought *you* were on.

on steps they might try to take in rehearsing a new dance in their relationship, or in their joint relationship with symptoms or illness.

Ten minutes for the couple

You saw Mrs B last week and invited her to make a double appointment with her husband. Just imagine that today she has mistakenly booked in for a 10-minute appointment. What can you possibly achieve in such a short time and what sort of map can you use to guide you? The consultation has a beginning, a middle and an end. In the first part you need to take a bit of a history, in the middle to explore the issues, and at the end come to some sort of resolution with possibly an agreed action plan. Relationship pain is like any other pain in the body. It has a history, it has exacerbating and relieving factors and it affects other parts of the body (in this case the family, friends and work). Couples use 'substances' like work, children, alcohol, hobbies amongst other things to forget about the pain. So, history taking should not be too much of a problem; narrowing down the consultation probably will be.

As a starting point you may find it useful to say 'As we have only 10 minutes and can tackle only one part of the problem, what do you both think is most important to discuss?' or perhaps 'What would make you feel that this consultation had been helpful?' If they say different things, you can follow up with: 'Would you like to talk about both of your important issues in this consultation or does one of you have a more pressing need than the other?' This gives you information about the power balance and problem-solving abilities of the relationship. If you sense that the wife is giving in to the husband's dominant narrative: 'Is it usual for your wife to defer to you in this way? If she disagreed would she be able to say so?' If your sense is that that they have come in to dump the problem on you: 'Supposing at the end of the consultation today one or other of you didn't find it helpful, who would you talk to instead? What else would you do?' This gives an idea that there may be other people more helpful and that the problem belongs to them.

If they start to have a row, you can let it continue for a little while – but not more than two minutes! Check out whether this is what happens at home (some people only argue in front of a referee!). If you think it is getting nowhere: 'Is this helpful to argue right now?' If yes: 'Can you explain what is helpful about arguing right now?' If no, suggest that they stop right away as it is a waste of time doing something unhelpful: 'So, if it's a waste of time, how could you now make good use of time? Please discuss that with each other.'

Summing up what has been discussed and agreed upon and deciding what should happen next is then in familiar territory for most clinicians.

Couple work and secrets

One fairly regular circumstance that arises in generalist practice is the 'Can-I-tell-you-something-and-can-you-pretend-I-didn't' scenario. 'I just want to tell you something important about Ahmed [husband] before he comes to see you today.' 'Could you come and see Mrs P? But please don't tell her I asked for you – she gets angry if I worry.' 'Can I just have a quick word?'

Now there are no hard and fast rules for this and there will certainly be circumstances where the clinician has no choice but to hold information and not attempt to enable more open and honest communication. You may be involved in separately helping both members of a divorcing couple. Simply holding the increasingly divergent stories of what is happening is both a skill we have to have and an object lesson in multiple 'truths' or realities. However, these 'opportunities for dissembling' or 'invitations to collude' can sometimes become opportunities to explore the nature of the relationship and decline to pretend or even lie to other patients. Being asked to share secrets that cannot then be talked about can seriously hamper your ability to be neutral or to perceive the different perspectives or stories of partners in a relationship. If you can see it coming or get your head in gear quickly enough you might like to try one or more of the following.

> PATIENT: *'I just want to tell you something important about Ahmed [husband] before he comes to see you today.'*

At this stage you need to both acknowledge that someone has taken the time to want to tell you something (and is invested in influencing the outcome of your upcoming meeting with Ahmed) but you need to see if you can get at the context in which you are being offered this information.

> CLINICIAN: *'I am glad you wanted to talk to me today and I am keen to hear what you want to tell me, but before you do, can I just check whether Ahmed knows you are going to tell me this? What would Ahmed think if he knew you were talking to me?'*

> PATIENT: *'Oh no – you mustn't tell Ahmed I told you this. He would be very upset if he knew I had told you.'*

So this is the crunch – do you simply accept this is part of the job or is it worth exploring whether there might be another way of getting this information into the public space between and with both partners? Sharing your dilemma can often be enough.

> CLINICIAN: *'I suspect this information is important to understanding how things are. But I would feel rather awkward knowing this and pretending I didn't know it. Do you see my problem?'*

> PATIENT: *'Well yes I can see that I suppose. It is just important for you to know.'*

There are a number of ways the clinician can go once you have slowed down the conversation enough for the patient to see that there are pros and cons to you hearing this information this way. The word to remember is 'pacing'. Find a way of taking time and not being hurried into decisions:

- 'Can I phone you back when I've had a think about what you have just said?'
- 'Have you asked Ahmed whether you can tell me this or explained why you feel this is so important for me to know about? Have you asked whether you could join him in seeing me? What would he say? What could you then say in order to help him see your point of view?'

- 'If you were to tell me this information and you were then to tell Ahmed you had done so – what would be the worse thing that could happen? Can you help me understand why Ahmed would be unhappy for you to tell me? What would he say if he was listening to this conversation now? Are there many areas where you would like to say things but can't? Do you think he also wants to tell me things but not want you to know about them?'
- 'Can you imagine what it would be like if I saw you both together?'

Now some of you at this point are thinking 'Life's too short – let's just hear what she has to say and then see where it takes us!' And that may be fine. You may be fearful that this is about some significant symptom which would clinch the diagnosis and you do not want to miss the opportunity to hear the information. Sometimes it may be fine to take the risk. But reflect on how many occasions accepting this information has hampered your ability to hear the partner's viewpoint or even to feel curious about the other person's 'take' on the issues. These 'gifts' can sometimes disempower you and ally you with a partner in ways that reduce you chances of staying neutral in the dance.

Couple work, lifestyle changes and health concerns

An increasing amount of your time in primary care is being spent discussing issues around lifestyle, risk and prevention, such as giving up smoking and weight reduction. Systemic thinking has a number of ideas to offer in this area. At the simplest level we are often enquiring about family history – specifically heart disease and other major illness. Recording this information on family trees is a very efficient way of capturing the data. But don't always leave it there! Occasionally you may be tempted to wonder aloud with the patient about what impact this has had on their way of thinking about life and death, about risk, about their attitudes to prevention or lifestyle change.

We suspect there is no reader of this book who has not heard a version of: 'Well, my Uncle Chang drank like a fish and smoked 30 unfiltered cigarettes a day – but he lived to be 95.' You can smile ruefully and continue burbling on about all the risks and the necessary changes your patient needs to make, or you could be more curious: 'So, do you feel you will be like your uncle? Are there other members of the family who had different experiences to Uncle Chang? – What is your understanding of this?'

Sometimes these conversations can liberate you both from the imposed tyranny of one of the most prevalent and powerful current cultural beliefs – that the object of life is to live as long as possible!

> PATIENT: 'Three score years and ten is what it says in the Bible – so anything over that is a bonus. I am 73 now – so it's all for fun from now on!'

> CLINICIAN [with relief]: 'Does that mean we don't need to talk about you smoking ever again?'

There is some evidence that working with couples rather than individuals around lifestyle change can be more effective (Doherty and Campbell 1988). People failing to lose weight often have partners who are critical of them, especially at meal times. This might arise because the partner is frightened that if the woman gets thinner she will leave him; on the other hand it might be for some other reason, like the fear they might be forced to eat rabbit food or solid meat as well!

Domestic violence

Domestic violence, a curiously sanitised notion for what it often hides, appears in primary care in a multitude of ways and is rarely addressed. Women may be depressed and not respond to antidepressants, they may have alcohol problems, sustain fractures, always appear at appointments with their partners. As domestic violence often appears for the first time during pregnancy and postnatally, many midwives and health visitors are now asking questions like:

- 'Does (or in the past has) anyone you know or love hurt you in any way physically, emotionally or sexually? I ask this question because it is so common for violence to begin in pregnancy.'
- 'Supposing it did happen in a month or two, how would you keep yourself safe? Who would you tell?'

To be bold and confident asking these sorts of questions the clinician needs to be familiar with the resources available locally. There is preventive work to be done in this area to help women keep themselves safe and enable men to understand their responsibility towards keeping their partners and children safe and also to understand the challenges for a man of the birth of his new baby. Of course, there is also some female-to-male violence – we are simply referring to the most common scenarios and the ideas apply equally well in other circumstances.

Supposing, as a health visitor, you visit a patient, knowing her partner 'has been a bit rough' the night before, because a neighbour has phoned the surgery to say so. How might you talk to the young mother on her own? Again clarity and straightforwardness helps.

Mrs B next door let me know that she heard Jim hitting you last night. Part of my job is to make sure you and the baby are safe. I'd like to talk to you about this and thought it might be helpful for you to listen to what I have to say and then let me know what you think.

 Parental history

In your next surgery try asking the three patients you don't know so well whether their parents are alive or dead and what they died of. Perhaps you could say: 'It strikes me I don't know much about your family history. Can you tell me a little about your parents?'

Then, rather than putting this info into a computer template, try one question exploring the impact of this information on your patient. 'I am curious. What impact did your mother's death when you were 18 have on you? Do you think it has influenced the way you feel about other aspects of your life?' This can be an interesting exercise in discovering about the beliefs that patients hold.

Explain that domestic violence is common (without minimising it by using language like 'getting a bit rough', 'a little shove'). Explain how difficult it can be to talk.

Supposing you knew it was going to happen again how would you make yourself safe? What would make it difficult? How can you make it easier to keep yourself safe? How safe are you having talked like this to me?

Further on down the line are the families where violence has been going on for years and the clinician feels despairing of anything ever changing. It takes very many episodes of violence, very many attempts at leaving (Goldner *et al.* 1990) to get out and stay out. Questions like:

- 'What did you learn when you left last time that helps you think more about keeping yourself safe? What do you think you will learn next time?'
- 'How will I know when you want me to help you to stay out of the relationship? How could I be most helpful to you then?'
- 'If it takes 27 episodes of violence for women to leave finally, how many episodes do you want to choose to go through? How could you manage to leave before that number was reached?'

The emphasis on neutrality is often helpful in this circumstance. It is very difficult to understand why people stay in violent relationships. Try asking the patient to help you understand what makes it difficult to leave or perhaps even asking what

Time out programmes

Time out programmes (van Lawick and Groen 1998) can be very effective, consisting of a number of steps:

1 The violent partner has to take responsibility for his acts, no matter what the 'provocations'.
2 Both partners are helped to identify and increase awareness of typical sequences leading to violent exchanges.
3 When one partner states 'danger' and asks for 'time out', the other is not allowed to argue or disagree with the request.
4 The person who takes 'time out' is also the person to make contact afterwards again.
5 Both partners reflect together on what should happen in practice:
   - where to go during 'time out'
   - how long for
   - how new contact is established after 'time out'
   - what to do with children
   - what to do when drugs or alcohol are involved.
6 The clinician discusses a variety of hypothetical scenarios to get each partner to think about possible actions and resolutions (e.g. middle of the night; in the car or in a public space; when visiting the extended family).

they find holds them in the relationship: 'Help me understand the things you value in your partner. When it is good what does he make you feel? Can you imagine doing without this feeling?'

It can also be an ideal time to look at the patient's own family issues. Often there has been violence or a pattern of intense emotions – both love and violence – from parents or other important figures in childhood. Tracing patterns, making them conscious, is a first step to breaking the cycle.

Conclusion

By inviting partners to attend, some 'live' action enters the consulting room. It allows for 'in vivo' observations to take place. It can also be very therapeutic if the clinician can get the couple to talk to one another about the things the patient previously felt could only be trusted to the clinician. However, it is not always easy to get both partners to attend simultaneously and this is why some 'courting' of the couple needs to take place first: the patient needs to be convinced to bring the partner, and then, in turn, to explore ways of convincing the partner to attend.

This work is not just confined to heterosexual partners; homosexual couples have similar – and some different – issues. The approach also lends itself to working with various other 'couples' who present with entrenched relationship problems, whether an octagenerian mother and her son in his sixties, an elderly brother and his sister living together, or any other combination.

 The 'couple factor'

1   Invite a suitable couple to attend for a slightly extended consultation. Pay attention to how you sell this idea to the presenting patient.

2   The next time you see more than one person in the surgery, encourage them to talk to one another about an issue they have brought up. Use phrases such as 'Can you talk to him about that now?' and 'Would you like to respond to that?' to get some 'live' (inter-)action in the consulting room. Record your observations about the consultation afterwards and identify areas of your own competence in conducting couple consultations. Evaluate your own position in relation to each partner and speculate about whose side each of them thought *you* were on.

3   Decide that on one day of next week you are going to research the 'couple factor' of every problem presented in surgery, from colds and blood pressure to terminal illness. Notice which questions you like and what different perspectives you get.

This chapter covers:
○   Convening family meetings
○   Orienting the family interview
○   Joining with the family
○   Practical skills for working with families
○   Enacting familiar problems
○   Anticipating and rehearsing new scenarios
○   Setting tasks
○   Using paradoxes

So far we have talked about bringing family members into the consultation as virtual members: drawing them in through genograms and circles, looping them in through questions, speculating with the individual about 'what if your father was here?' 'What would your daughter say?'. Then in the previous chapter we introduced some skills for working with couples in primary care, but there are also times when it is worth the effort and time required to bring more than two people into the room at once. In this chapter we want to work with the family 'in the flesh'. Although this chapter is primarily about families, the skills learnt here also lend themselves to other multi-person meetings – network meetings, case conferences and care programme approach (CPA) meetings.

Why, how and when to convene families

It is unlikely that planning and convening a family will be an everyday occurrence, but it probably happens occasionally already. Sometimes both parents collect all their children, including the ill one, and rush down to the surgery after school hours. At other times you might walk into a patient's home to find a family assembled around a poorly patient's bedside. These spontaneous crisis family meetings can be remarkably exciting and rewarding when you are up to the challenge (see the next chapter for more details). However, much more often the idea and organisation for a family meeting will need to come from you. So when is it appropriate to work this way? Perhaps the simplest answer is whenever it feels that a patient's difficulty involves the family in a significant and ongoing way and particularly where this involvement is leading to further difficulties.

Thinking families in severe or chronic illness

There will be occasions when you wish to try some initial work with a family around predominantly psychological issues – terrible arguing, mental health problems, imminent divorce. But how about the huge area of families working with 'physical' illness? Families have a significant impact on the life history of illness and illness, as you all know, has a significant effect on the family.

Here are some specific occasions when meeting with the family might be really helpful:

- New and significant illness has been diagnosed, such as severe and acute illness (e.g. heart attack or subarachnoid haemorrhage) or cancer.
- A chronic or life-threatening illness, such as Parkinson's disease or Alzheimer's, has been diagnosed.
- A child is presented with behavioural or emotional problems, such as sleep difficulties, eating and feeding problems, tantrums, adolescent crises, drug and alcohol problems, challenging teenagers.

There are, of course, myriads of points in time when other family members are suddenly more closely involved in a particular patient's story. And often this is entirely without problem or issue. There is an illness or crisis, and members of the family respond; support and care is given; the situation resolves or the family adapts and continues in ways that allow individual members to function successfully. Long-standing social institutions like families are, in many cultures, hugely successful and stable units for most people most of the time, even if the forms of family structure are now more varied than previously. However, there are plenty of times when the balance of a family is perturbed, the gyroscope wobbles more precariously, the steps of the dance get lost or so ingrained that no other steps are possible. Some families are like that – those are the steps and odd though it may appear to some, that's how they do it. Some families learn to shout, and shouting is OK! Others never learn that and then, if someone does shout, it is definitely NOT OK! Older ideas about the 'right' way for families to function and, by implication, the 'wrong' way have faded as attempts have been made to see what works and what does not. There are certainly many families where it is not working so well and it is then that clinicians need to be more curious and wonder whether taking the family focus would pay off.

Meeting the family – 'invitations to the ball' and 'bouncers at the door'

Creating the opportunity to talk with Mrs N about her heart attack along with her elderly husband and the daughter that lives at home with them can seem a good one. But how to make it happen? Sometimes going to the patient's house can make the logistics of meeting whole families simpler. It can reduce formality and allows the clinician to meet the family more on its own terms. Health visitors and district nurses are ideally placed to see families this way. But GPs can find that asking to see the family, or as much of it as can be brought together, is achieved more easily by asking to meet at the house. And for space reasons at many practices this may also be more practical. Psychiatry for the Elderly services often visit patients at home – a very welcome development. The slow realisation that a partner is dementing can be one of the hardest family adjustments to make. Wouldn't it be excellent if there was time to have both the psychiatric nurse and a primary care clinician meet with the family? And perhaps sometimes setting that up would be cost effective as roles and expectations are clarified and generalist and specialist 'knowledges' and support are combined with family resilience.

Next please ...

Mr and Mrs E are well known to the practice: Mr E for all his good charity works and Mrs E for her diabetes and failure to keep appointments. Their adult children are always on the phone asking for this, that and the other. When Mr E was diagnosed with cancer all hell broke loose in the team (and probably in specialist care!). The numbers of phone calls quadrupled as the family demanded instant and simultaneous access to all four GPs, the physician, the surgeon and the oncologist. The daughter phoned and harangued the new principle for breaking the bad news to her parents before she knew, saying she wanted to be involved in all decisions. She told the new GP she thought she was inexperienced and callous in the way she had handled things, having told the receptionists the same story.

Mr and Mrs E were invited in to talk about how they would like their care to be managed. The GP explained the way the practice would like to do this, by having two doctors knowing what was going on so that they got consistent feedback and continuity. She explained that it was the practice's job to help the family manage their crisis in the way that they wanted and not to impose ideas on them.

The family were Irish Catholic living in a city in northern England. They said they were very close and wanted everyone to be kept informed. The GP recognised that their behaviour in Ireland would have been viewed as normal. She commented (thinking positively!) on how their daughter seemed to be showing how she cared by phoning and wanting to be involved. They agreed and said it was all the more remarkable because their daughter's marriage had just broken up and most women in her situation wouldn't have had the energy to bother. They were very proud of her. As the weeks went on various family members formed a close relationship with the practice, never missed appointments and were polite to the receptionists, who were amazed at the power of a crisis to transform people's behaviour. Their perception had been that the wife wouldn't be able to cope with the burden of caring.

If you are intending to work more proactively with a family at home it is important, however, to make sure you have successfully negotiated agreement about the benefit of the meeting. Professionals are powerful – even if they themselves do not perceive themselves in that way – and they can often hold their views about the benefit of meetings despite clear anxieties to the contrary. Many of the techniques for exploring the utility of a couple meeting apply just as much to family meetings. So watch your power! Having said that, it is worth bearing in mind the following quote:

It must be considered that nothing is more difficult to carry out, nor more doubtful of success, nor more dangerous to handle, than to initiate a new order of

things. For the reformer has enemies in all those who profit by the old order, and only the lukewarm defenders in all those who would profit by the new order . . . who do not truly believe in anything new until they have actual experience of it.
(Machiavelli 1469–1527)

Sometimes it is worth pushing quite hard. After all, families that do not want to change will be little damaged by your efforts, whereas those that do, may well appreciate the chance!

Invitations to the ball

Usually the venue for the meeting will be the practice. Whether a meeting at the family's home or at the practice is planned, the first task is to invite family members to the ball. Many of the principles we talked about when inviting a partner apply equally here.

- 'One of the things I like to offer in this situation is to meet with more of the family.'
- 'Often I find meeting with other family members can be very helpful at a time like this.'
- 'It seems to me that this problem/illness/situation is not only affecting you but also other members of the family. How would it be if we were to get them to join us to talk it through?'

And even

- 'I am not sure how much more I can offer in this situation without getting other members of the family in to help us.'

Bouncers at the door

Many of the barriers and hurdles to meeting with the family will be similar to those with the couple (see Chapter 9) and many of the techniques for moving a person towards the idea will be similar too. Issues of risk, confidentiality, secrets, as well as cultural and family beliefs may all be significant barriers. Understanding these barriers may well be therapeutic in itself and may then lead to a greater confidence in the idea of working with the family.

Working with families – 'putting on your dancing shoes'

As you know by now, one of our favourite metaphors for systemic practice is that of the 'dance'. Most dances are interlocking patterns of steps and gestures taken by two or more people. The steps fit together, are frequently rehearsed, practised and learnt by memory and are often very familiar. Much of human interaction can usefully be seen as a dance. Do you know the 'Distancer–pursuer two-step'? Have you heard of the 'Status quo' and 'All-change partnership tango'? The 'Partner twist and shout'? The 'Old age slow trot'? Have you watched and been confused by the whirling of an 'Eightsome reel' and enjoyed the gentle repetition of 'Strip the willow'? The best ceilidhs manage to incorporate even the most inexperienced dancers with ease. Perhaps this is the vision a newly family-minded clinician should have in mind. Elegant experienced eightsomes are all very well, but they just aren't as much fun.

Many consultations can be seen as a dance. You will all be familiar with those patients who repeatedly come to see you but with no resolution to their problems. Despite your best efforts – or maybe because of them – things always seem to turn out the same as before. These repetitive patterns can sometimes be a curious source of pleasure for both parties as you again take your positions for another 'No change waltz', but more often they are a source of frustration. One role of the clinician in a family consultation is to offer the occasional different step, to encourage patients to try out a different dance, tempting someone to experiment with a new routine. Of course, even one 'new' or 'wrong' step can be enough to upset the usual pattern – brief periods of uncertainty may ensue before the family settles into a new dance, hopefully with steps more to their mutual liking. The clinician sets the key in the hope that the family will tune in and 'move'. Some families wish to play their own tunes and control the entire interview. Whichever way it is, getting the family to establish its own rhythms and motifs must be the major aim of family consultation, with the clinician occasionally slowing down or quickening the pace, at times stopping the tune altogether or introducing a new 'step', or variation, to get the family to experiment with something new.

Inviting the whole family to attend at the surgery is a more formal event than meeting its members at a domiciliary visit. It is different in that the clinician has requested the family to come, and it is therefore up to the clinician to introduce

Dance spotting

In five minutes see how many repetitive patterns you can identify:

*   in your own close relationships
*   within the partnership or practice in which you work.

Think of the times someone has wanted change, when something has gone wrong, when you want something of the other person, when you are stressed, when you are happy.

Have a think about how many of these dances feel familiar, and reflect on how difficult it is to change the steps!

Finally, you might like to think about the dances you have with particular patients:

*   When you become the couple's arbitrator
*   When you are a surrogate mother or son
*   When you seem to be the family punchbag or dustbin
*   When you are the anxiety regulator
*   When you try to 'glue' the couple together.

Share your findings with a few colleagues – and watch their steps!

and give the family meeting an 'orientation'. This provides a map within which to dance and sets the clinician as a careful choreographer:

> *Hello [shakes everyone's hands]. Thank you for coming. I have asked you all to come here today as a family. I thought this might be a good idea so that I can understand how each of you see Mrs Y's problem and how it affects everyone. And this may help Mrs Y to get better.*

In this way the reason given for the family meeting is to help the patient, rather than to give the family a good grilling, or blame them for the ill-health of the patient. It begins to make it safe for the family to dance. It is important to explain things in this or similar ways because many families will be somewhat puzzled by the clinician's request for all of them to come to the surgery. Many families indeed arrive with certain fears and trepidations, particularly when one member has already been to see the clinician: 'What did she tell the doctor?' 'Is he blaming us?'

Preparing the 'ballroom'

The ballroom needs enough chairs even for 3-year-olds lest the dance becomes musical chairs! If the family is seen within normal surgery hours, then there needs to be clarity with the reception staff about interruptions. Just as the room needs to be prepared, so do some family members. It is helpful for the clinician to have raised the following question with the patient prior to the first family meeting: 'How much of what we have been talking about may I share with the rest of the family. Or would you rather tell them yourself at the first meeting?'

In the first family meeting the clinician can open with the following statement: 'Mrs A, we have met before without the family and discussed some problems. Would you like to tell them about what we said – or would you like me to say and you can correct me if I've got it wrong?' This should signal to attending family members that the clinician is only human – and that he or she might get it wrong and is happy about being put right. It also conveys that the clinician has an open mind and that there is no one truth or absolute certainty – and this applies to family members as well as clinicians. Usually everyone is apprehensive at the beginning of a family meeting, with the clinician being no exception. If this is one of the first times the clinician has conducted a family interview, the sheer number of people in the room – and the raw emotions displayed by one or more of them – can feel intimidating.

To turn the family meeting into a special event, the clinician may consider using a different room: this makes it feel different, but also it is different for the family members who are then in a new and unfamiliar setting, different from the one in which they usually consult the clinician. Different contexts often elicit different behaviours.

Joining the family – the introductory bow

We have chosen to think about a family with younger children in it as this is a common pattern you may see. Most of the principles still apply to families where all are adult. The most important step is to 'join' (Minuchin 1974) with all family members. This is crucial, as some relatives may not be well known to you and others may feel, rightly or wrongly, that you are on the index patient's side. The term 'joining' means to make a connection with each member of the family, to form a therapeutic alliance, to let them know that you want to understand them. You can join with patients in all sorts of ways – a first step is to get the family to introduce everyone:

> *I know we have, one way or another, all met at some point but I would like you to help me to remember names and ages. Maybe each of you could say a few words about the person sitting next to you. Shall we go round clockwise? Who would like to start?*

This is one way of getting the ball rolling. Family members may not know who should start and the ensuing discussion gives you the opportunity to study how the family makes decisions, even apparently trivial ones. If they get stuck then you may wish to rescue the family by suggesting that either father or mother should start. *How* each person introduces the one sitting next to them can be full of surprises and gives first glimpses of live family dynamics. One aim of having the whole family there is to see how they interact as individuals.

The next step is to engage briefly with each person directly. It is often best to begin with the youngest member of the family so that they feel included right from the start. Children can sometimes get restless and disruptive and make the interview quite difficult, but if they are engaged with in the first few minutes their attention is more likely to be won for the rest of the meeting. Making contact with young children is usually not very difficult, you can ask them about school, their interests, friends – and perhaps why they think that they had to come with the family to the surgery.

The opening tune

> *Mr and Mrs Y, I would like to talk to Jasmin and ask her a few questions. Is that all right? If there is anything I shouldn't ask her, please let me know – or if indeed you don't want her to answer, please tell her. The last thing I want to do is to make things awkward for anyone.*

This seemingly long-winded preamble is necessary and usually puts parents at ease: first, they are being asked their permission for the clinician to interview their child. Second, they are asked to veto, if necessary, certain questions or answers. In other words, it puts responsibility onto the parents to be in charge of the overall flow of the interview, and indirectly their children, so that it cannot later be claimed that the clinician made things worse for the children by asking embarrassing or seem-ingly 'harmful' questions. It is of course possible to ask apparently innocuous questions which address issues that the parents would rather not be discussed and it is therefore most important to give parents overall control over the interview. In this way parental rights and authority can be respected.

If the clinician becomes disconnected from one or more family members the interview will become more difficult as their attention lapses or as they feel unim-portant. It is important to remain connected with every member of the family, by looking at each for equivalent amounts of time, and by listening and talking to all members even-handedly. If 'meaty' issues arise with one member, then it is tempting to chase these issues and to forget to remain connected with the remaining members of the family. If you asked each family member at the end of a family meeting whose side they thought you were on, then they should say 'on nobody's' or, better still, 'on everybody's'!

So why do you think you are here?

One good way of focusing on the problem is to ask each family member, from the youngest child upwards, what he or she believes is the reason for the whole family attending: 'Why do you think you all came here as a family today?' or 'What did your mum and dad explain to you about coming here?' Then 'If you don't know, do you want to ask them now? [to parents] Is it alright if she asks you now?' In this way, communication between family members in the consultation is encouraged. It often happens that a parent steps in and answers on the child's behalf, or that a brother or sister is disruptive. Such family interactions and processes are important sources of information: they demonstrate how the different members of the family talk to one another, how they support or disqualify one another, how roles are allocated, who is the spokesperson for the family, and so on. Again it is important to make sure everyone has the chance to say why they think they have come. If the family hold six different reasons for coming or six whole separate problems, then your work may simply be in narrowing down to a manageable conversation. Asking members to help you with this is often a good way of saying metaphorically: ' I am not solving all this. It's up to you to try and decide what would be most useful to talk about and if you can't decide then maybe we need to talk about how difficult it is to decide things.'

Another way would be to go back to the index patient and ask for their guidance as to where to start.

What is next?

After this opening there will be some pressure on the clinician to be in charge of the interview and it may now be important to ask circular and reflexive questions (see Chapter 4) about how each family member sees the illness or problem, and to speculate about its causes and the effects on the various family members. There is, however, one important additional feature about asking these questions when the whole family is present: instead of asking each person what they themselves think about the problem and its effects, it is often more useful to ask it indirectly: 'How do you, Jasmin, think your father is affected by your mother's illness?' This way of questioning is called *triadic*: it elicits information about how a third person sees the relationship between two others. It is a sort of professional form of gossiping. Family clinicians would do well to squash the old phrase 'two's company, three's none'. To systemic practitioners, two's company and three is fascinating. In threes you can see alliances, when family members form partnerships and coalitions, with two people ganging up against a third. Such alliances and coalitions 'move' round the room in a supple family – and are rooted to the floor in stuck families.

Asking triadic questions is a potentially provocative approach in that the two people present about whom the third person communicates, will respond to it, agreeing or disagreeing. Even if it is not put into words at this point, later on, after the consultation, individual family members may challenge one another about what each said. Triadic questions encourage people to mind-read in the presence of others who cannot help but respond to these (true or false) assumptions. Such an interview can be therapeutic in itself in that it helps people to see things differently and make new connections. It brings out into the open disagreements and conflicts that have been hidden previously and thus is a first step to sorting things out. For example, 'I never knew you thought that was what I thought!' 'Why did you think I would think that?' New light from different directions makes things look different. That may be enough to cause a family to start to act differently.

Enacting familiar problems – demonstrating the steps

Getting two or more people to 'enact the problem' (Minuchin 1974) is often a good way of observing family interaction and gives glimpses of the problematic behaviours. Such enactments are set up deliberately: the clinician asks for the 'trouble' to be demonstrated 'in vivo'! Here are some ways of setting up enactments: 'Let me see what it is that you have to do or say for Jasmin to have the sort of temper tantrum that you find so difficult to cope with. What would you have to do or say now?' or 'Perhaps you and your husband could think now about an issue that you feel you might have an argument about . . . maybe money, the children, mother-in-law . . . what would you have to say to get him or her going?' or ask another member of the family 'What do mum and dad mostly argue about? Can you suggest their favourite topic to them?'

It is surprising how well people know which 'button' to press to make happen what they so often claim they have 'no control whatsoever' over their family members. Knowing how to make things happen is the first step to considering what *not* to do so that these things do not happen! When such an enactment happens it can become quite heated and the clinician may intensify things further by saying, for example,

> *Your little girl seems to be winning. Do you want her to win again? Do you want her to beat you all the time? So if you don't, why don't you show her*

Connections between ideas about change

The creation of new perspectives is an activity most therapeutic approaches have in common. Psychodynamic therapists use transference interpretations, pointing out how the patient projects aspects of themselves onto the therapist. This provides a new view and 'insight' for the patient. Cognitive behavioural therapists ask patients to examine their beliefs and other cognitions, encouraging them to look at themselves from another point of view. Some yogis practise 'astral projection', viewing themselves and their interactions from a virtual bird's eye perspective. Working with families permits the introduction of yet further perspectives – that of each family member, in addition to the 'frames' the therapist provides.

that you are the boss, that she cannot get away with blackmailing you. Show her now, I'll sit back and let you get on with it.

Such an approach requires the clinician's belief that parents will find their own resources if encouraged. They may turn repeatedly to the clinician and ask for advice: 'What shall I do now?' If this advice is not immediately forthcoming the parents need to get into discussion with one another how to best handle this 'crisis' situation. Often it becomes apparent that there is disagreement between them, usually one being the 'soft' and the other the 'tough' one. The clinician's intervention then is fairly straightforward:

How can you expect your Jasmin to know what to do, if she hears 'stereo'. Mother says one thing and dad says another thing. Each is very sensible, but both together must be confusing to her, particularly if she knows that you will be the 'toughie' and you will be the 'softie'. Is she so tough because you are so soft, or are you so soft because she is so tough? Can you both now talk to each other so that you can then talk to your daughter with one voice rather than two – otherwise she'll get very confused.

This intervention can be extremely effective. The family has enacted the problem in the room, and based on these live observations the clinician is able to describe how both parents are giving incongruent and inconsistent messages to their daughter. How the two behaviours complement one another can then be addressed by implying that mother's softness may be the response to father's real or alleged toughness, and vice versa. The clinician then encourages the parents to come together and join forces so that their daughter can receive a 'straight' message. Another option is to ask the parents to swap roles or to think about swapping roles. What would the mother like about being tough if she knew dad would be soft? What would she dislike? What would dad find the advantages and disadvantages of being soft for a change?

Next please . . .

In one family seen by the practice psychologist, a lively 8-year-old school-refusing boy was given the task of being his own mother and trying to persuade 'this little boy', in a mini role play, to go to school. Mother role-played the boy. They had little difficulty in doing so. After five minutes they were asked to sit back and comment on the experience. Mother said that she had really enjoyed being argumentative and 'naughty'. The boy found that being his mother was hard work: 'When I was mum, I really hated this little brat . . . eh me.' The psychologist asked if it was important to continue these battles. 'It's fun to have arguments', said the boy, 'But not about school' added the mother. The psychologist then asked them to think about other things they could safely argue about as arguing might be very important and 'character forming' for the boy. Both laughed and then had a mock argument about whether it was going to rain or not that day.

Such enactments are very intense experiences for families (and clinicians!) and usually stay with them once they have left the surgery. The next time a similar situation occurs at home, the parents and child(ren) will remember how things evolved in front of the clinician and build on the experiences from the 'dress-rehearsal', hopefully changing the steps of an all too familiar dance routine.

Anticipating and rehearsing – trying new steps: 'practice makes perfect'

Let us assume that there has been a successful enactment and resolution of a typical problem in the surgery. The clinician can then get the family to anticipate the next similar event and rehearse their responses. To do this, the family could be asked:

- 'What are you going to do the next time this happens? Who is going to do what?'
- 'I now want you to predict when this next time is. Today? Tomorrow? At what time? What are you going to do Mr X? And what about you Mrs X?'
- 'Would it perhaps be better if I prescribed a crisis for you, so that you can have a chance to put into practice what you've tried here? Oh, you don't need that – well, can you then engineer your own crisis and talk about how you're going to resolve it?'

Most patients are able to predict specific crises with accuracy. To do this in a hypothetical situation with the patient(s) may be very helpful, particularly when it results in new ways of anticipating and preventing such crises: 'So when that happens what can you do differently? What is Y's response going to be? Do you want that to happen? So what would you have to do differently for that not to happen?'

Crisis points can be imagined and new strategies rehearsed: 'Imagine you and X are in that situation. You know something is going to explode anytime now. What are you going to do differently?' The clinician could, for brief moments, assume the role of one of the participants, like a devil's advocate, and provoke the family to experiment with new solutions to familiar problems: 'What if she gets angry and shouts at you: "You never support me"?' or 'What if he withdraws and says in a miserable voice: "Nobody loves me"?'

Homework tasks – dancing without your coach

Encouraging families to have (predictable) crises is a bit like giving them some homework. This can be particularly useful if it arises naturally out of a family consultation as it is then built on some strong experience they have already had in the consulting room. Transferring such learning into the home will generalise the effects. In this way families have to think about specific issues and experiment with different behaviours after the consultation. This implies that therapy is not simply dished out by the clinician in the surgery, but that the family itself can become responsible for the healing process by doing things between consultations. To this end tasks can be prescribed that relate in some way to the presenting problem or aim at altering certain interactions that may result in symptomatic improvement.

One such task is to get the parent(s) or a whole family to record problematic or symptomatic behaviours prospectively: 'I would like you to keep a diary and make some observations about Mrs X's depression and record these for one week. Record the time it occurs, who is around when it happens, what the various people do and the outcome.'

A variation on this theme is to encourage each parent or partner to keep separate diaries and compare notes after one week. This puts family members (which could of course include children) into the role of observers in relation to their own family life. As the observer is part of the field of the observed it will inevitably affect normal processes in the family. These and other observations can then provide the 'material' for the next consultation. This homework can come to life if the family members are asked to be anthropologists 'finding out how aggression is managed in the X family'. Alternatively, someone could be a journalist trying to find out what every member of the extended family thinks about cross words being used. The choice of 'occupation' depends very much on the preferences expressed by the family.

Next please . . .

A 7-year-old boy couldn't tolerate his mother saying 'No' and would throw massive tantrums. He was mad about football and so he was asked to imagine himself as a goalkeeper and his mother scoring a goal each time he lost his cool when she said 'No'. She would warn him by saying 'Penalty shoot-out', he would catch the 'No' and then talk about it with his father when he returned from work.

Other tasks can be tailor-made to suit a particular family's structure:

*   A quarrelling husband and wife could be asked to have a romantic dinner once a week.
*   A conflict-avoiding couple could be prescribed one row per day after the children have gone to bed.
*   A distant father and son could be encouraged to spend more time with one another engaged in an activity they both enjoy.

The point of giving such tasks is to get patients and families to experiment with doing things differently and then see how that affects their relationships. The clinician should not be too prescriptive, but make light of the tasks and state that it is entirely up to the family to carry these out or not.

So you are all together to watch Eastenders? *OK, so after that you might wish to turn the telly off and then discuss, as a family, how you each feel about one another. Everyone has five minutes to say his or her bit, not a minute longer. Nobody should be allowed to respond immediately, people should just take turns in speaking and being heard. Once everyone has had their say, there should be silence for five minutes and then everyone can say what they want or leave. You can do this if you want to and it might be useful but it is entirely up to you. You won't get good or bad marks from me if you do.*

Change is difficult for everyone. By encouraging families to consider making very minor changes in the way they do things, they may get the experience of accomplishing a task and a first taste of progress and success. To be successful, tasks must be concrete and instructions precise.

Parents 'stepping out'

One particularly effective intervention, which needs to be used carefully, is the prescription of disappearing acts, which can lead to dramatic resolutions, particularly in enmeshed families with older children and younger adults. In these families the parents are often very anxious about separations and this makes the maturational process for their teenagers difficult. The way it was originally used by the Milan School of family therapy is probably now inappropriate, but it is still useful.

> *If you had been seen by some very famous Italian therapists about 20 years ago, you would've been involved in a routine they developed for managing these problems that was highly successful for crazy teenage behaviour. Would you like to hear about it? I have to say that I couldn't be as bossy as they were because I like to let people take charge of their own decision making about family situations. But it worked time after time so there must be some ingredients which are very important. They used to make parents promise to do exactly what they were told without telling them what they were agreeing to! They then told them to disappear for a few hours or an evening leaving a message that they were safe but didn't know when they would return. No one else was allowed to know where they were.*

This has the effect of a pebble dropped in a pond making ripples. You then observe the responses and comment, getting the parents to elaborate on their reactions: 'I notice that you are smiling, I wonder what is amusing you.' Parents will some-times say that it would be fun to give the teenagers a dose of their own medicine, but then say they would feel guilty for not setting a good example. You can then explain that they are being responsible because they are adults leaving a clear, safe message and a challenge to the adolescent to manage the situation themselves.

They often then begin to say that they are looking forward to the freedom of being a parent with children who have left home. This can then lead onto a more future-oriented discussion about life after children and the clinician can get more of a picture of underlying marital satisfaction by judging the enthusiasm with which the future is embraced. Normalising the life cycle tasks of re-establishing the couple relationship at this time can be helpful. Talking like this helps to put a boundary around the parental marital relationship which aids in the separation process. Talking to them about their experiences of being teenagers and leaving home helps them to compare the processes over generations. Many parents realise that they are exploring a territory with no map, which is understandably anxiety provoking. Some parents respond with a look of horror and state that they could not possibly do this, being worried about how other relatives and friends might react. The clinician can help by getting them to consider the following questions, in anticipation of some of the issues likely to be raised:

- 'How would you explain to your parents what you are doing?'
- 'How would you like them to respond when your son phones to complain? What difference would it make keeping it secret from your parents?'
- 'What are your worst fears about doing this?'
- 'Are these fears more or less likely to come about if you carry on doing as you are?'
- 'Imagine that as a result of you disappearing without warning, your son surprised you with his responsibility. How would that influence the decision you make now?'
- 'Supposing he was upset, but you were determined this was the right course of action. How might you respond to him?'
- 'How might his reactions change each time you repeated this disappearance act? How long would it be before he got used to the idea?'

At the end of the interview it is helpful to say:

> *We have explored a lot of interesting ideas. I wonder if you could go away and talk about one of these 'Italian' ingredients that has struck you as being worth trying as an experiment. Then you can report back to me the good and bad points of your experiment next time we meet.*

Indirect challenging

Primary health care workers can usually not afford to side with one patient at the expense of other family members. It is quite possible that the next day the spouse or granny will need to be seen for unrelated medical problems. If the clinician has been perceived as being 'grossly unfair', this may make a subsequent consultation more difficult if not impossible. However, at times it is very important to challenge people's assumptions and behaviours. Instead of going on a head-on collision course, a less confrontational yet challenging approach can be most useful. Indirect challenging can take the form of telling the family about 'some other patients' (real or imagined), obviously concealing their real identity in an attempt to talk about a 'parallel' story or predicament to help patients to connect with certain consequences of 'no change'. For example:

> *Some years ago I saw a boy aged three. His parents said he was 'out of control'. They said they never disciplined him, and they believed that he would grow out of it. They refused help at that point. I later learned that at six this boy was a professional blackmailer and bullied other kids at school. At nine he was caught shoplifting for the first time. At 11 he knifed his mother, at 16 he had already spent 10 months in a borstal. Somehow these parents had waited for too long. Of course, this was a very different family from yours, and your son is only three now.*

Another way of introducing anxiety-provoking information is to distance yourself from it: 'If I was a really bad clinician, I would say . . .' (and then you can say something challenging).

Focusing on just one topic is another way of indirectly challenging the way people habitually communicate with one another. Often couples or families appear to be unable to stick to one small problem or topic. Keeping a tight focus can be a way of forcing families to look at issues in some considerable detail and challenging any avoidance of dealing with such issues: 'Could you just come back to this for a minute. I agree, all these other issues are also very important, but if you don't resolve one issue, however small, it is unlikely that you are going to resolve all the others' or 'I find it impossible to discuss more than one issue at a time, so can we agree when we move on to the next topic.'

There are many other ways in which the clinician can disrupt or block dysfunctional communications. For instance, it may work to just draw attention to the process evolving in front of you: 'I notice you all talk at the same time – is that helpful to you all?' or 'May I stop you for a minute. Would it be OK for me to suggest that you, Mr X, should now listen for the next two minutes without interrupting your wife. And afterwards you can do it the other way round. Let's see whether that gets you anywhere.'

Summing up and messages

Many clinicians want to end a family consultation by summing up and possibly giving a message to the family. Such a message usually points out how everyone appears to want to help: 'The fact that you all came here today shows me that you all want to help and that is a very good thing.'

Many families feel criticised by professionals and parents cannot help blaming themselves for the problems their offspring present. It is therefore most important for clinicians to acknowledge the strengths and resources of the family and each individual member. The clinician can thank the family again for attending and state that it is up to them whether to carry out the task(s) prescribed or not. At this point it is useful to ask the family to decide whether they want to have another appointment. Often there is no immediate agreement amongst family members and this gives another opportunity to study the family interaction. It is instructive to note how decisions are arrived at and who has the final say. If there is time pressure the clinician could ask the family to get back once an agreement has been reached.

Paradoxical interventions

Patients and their families can sometimes find themselves in situations that seem painful or uncomfortable. Even though common sense might suggest that a change from such an unpleasant situation would be a good idea, paradoxically some people appear to 'prefer' being miserable to apparently being relieved of some stress, particularly when the alternatives seem more threatening. For example, it may be more comfortable to drown one's sorrows regularly in alcohol rather than to confront them. Moreover, many spouses collude with the excessive drinking as it can suit them as well. In this way the alcohol becomes some kind of 'medication', keeping things – and people – subdued. Often the (imagined) alternative pains of confrontation, separation and loneliness seem so much worse. This then explains why any attempts to challenge or change the alcohol-related behaviour can encounter tremendous resistance.

Paradoxical interventions (Selvini Palazzoli *et al.* 1978) usually positively connote the problem and encourage the patient or family to continue with the symptom and related behaviours, thereby prescribing the symptom: 'Sometimes there are very good reasons why people just don't get better. For instance, getting better can seem like opening a can of worms. So before you consider changing anything it is important to weigh up the pros and cons for you and your family.'

Learning to create the symptoms/behaviours can be a powerful way of learning about them and how to control them: 'Supposing I asked you to deliberately go and drink too much now, how would you set about it to make your wife most upset?' 'Supposing you decided you didn't want to do what I had said, how would you ensure that that didn't happen?'

Sometimes what is needed when patients seem to resist our best endeavours is to think of a different way of understanding the problem. Is it our problem or theirs? 'Supposing nothing changed for you and you stayed feeling 5 out of 10 about your family situation, how long would that be OK to go on for? What would have to happen to make you want to come back and think differently about things?'

Paradoxes should be used very sparingly in primary health care, usually as a last resort or when patients appear to be fighting all the clinician's attempts to get them better. Paradoxes should not be used in cases of family violence, sexual abuse, parasuicide, death and normal grief situations, or unwanted pregnancies. Above all it is important to deliver paradoxical interventions sensitively, in such a way that families do not feel ridiculed. Here are some examples:

> *I accept that you have come here because of X [symptom] which is very upsetting or painful to you. Of course you would like to get rid of X as quickly as possible. Desirable though this may seem at first sight, there are dangers in changing this dramatically because it might disturb the equilibrium of the family. I would therefore like to suggest that for the time being you should continue doing X and only stop when you decide that the family no longer needs you to do this.*

Next please . . .

Mr and Mrs B have endless rows and seem reluctant to give these up. The practitioner may give them the following 'advice':

   'It does seem that the rows have gone on for a long time and they seem to have become part of your way of life. I do not expect you to stop and, in fact, would be a bit worried if you did. What I would like to suggest is:

1   *that at no time do you become physically violent*
2   *that if you begin to have a row, you move into the hall before you continue it*
3   *that you each imagine what outside observers, such as myself, would see if they were present*
4   *that you record your observations for each row afterwards, which, if you want to, you can bring here for discussion.'*

Here the clinician is not discouraging rows, but asks the couple to have them in a different, almost ritualised context, as well as becoming the observers of these events. When prescribing modified paradoxes for patients presenting with physical symptoms, the clinician apparently accepts the patient's illness position:

- *'Given that we have agreed that it might be dangerous to change anything at present, how often should we meet to discuss it?'*
- *'Given that nothing is changing, what are the most helpful questions for me to ask when I see you?'*
- *'If I were being more helpful, what would I be saying or doing? At the moment I feel quite helpless.'*

This may force a family or patient to assume a counter position, namely encouraging the clinician not to give up and showing some positive changes so as to keep him or her involved in the 'dance'. A new step for the clinician to take is to move from 'treating the patient' to 'monitoring the situation' on a regular basis, possibly even hinting that any other involvement might interfere with the healing process. Paradoxical? Hardly – particularly if we take account of iatrogenic and other unwanted side effects often accompanying the interventions of keen clinicians.

Conclusion

All these techniques, from triadic questions to way-out paradoxes, are designed to change some of the steps in the family dance, to perturb the family's painful equilibrium. They are nudges to put people just a little off balance – to provide new perspectives and try out new steps. Real lasting change does not happen in the consulting room, it mostly happens afterwards. The consultation is simply a vehicle encouraging and empowering families to change direction.

Some techniques described in this chapter may seem rather provocative – challenging the status quo. Maybe that is why they should carry an 'Authors' Enthusiasm Warning': 'Family work can change your (or the family's) health.'

For many readers, convening and conducting formal family meetings with unhappy, poorly functioning or distressed families is going to be a relatively rare event. It can be enormously rewarding and if you can find a friendly ally in the form of a local family-trained specialist and there is room in the practice then this sort of work can be a very welcome addition to the practice services. However, it will not be possible for many of you for a whole variety of reasons.

What is possible, desirable and much more do-able is to see families or bits of families when there are specific crises – deaths, illnesses, particular ways of coping with problems or events. The skills we have outlined above will all be useful in those circumstances. How to work with families in crisis is the subject of the next chapter.

 ## Conclusions

1. *Orientation* Think of a time when you were not prepared properly for what was to follow (a small operation, interview, etc.). How should you have been prepared? What did the dance feel like to you? Who should have choreographed the steps?

2. *Joining* Notice what happens when someone is not introduced properly. Have a think about how new team members are inducted to the practice. Who should you talk to about these observations?

3. *Become an anthropologist* Research why changing your clinical behaviour is difficult. Choose three of the techniques from this chapter that appeal to your style of consulting and try them out. Ask the patients what they thought of your new approach. Who else might you talk to about the results of this research? Which responses would you like most – and least?

4. Think of a situation at work with your team that made you feel furious. Find at least three *positive reframes* for what happened.

The family in crisis 11

This chapter covers:
- ○ A template for thinking about crises
- ○ Systemic practice and crisis prevention
- ○ Families' crisis coping strategies
- ○ Coping strategies for primary care teams in crisis

If you were to look back over the previous week's consultations, how many would you have considered were being triggered by crises? The diagnosis of gastric cancer in a 45-year-old man, or the potential suicide risk of a depressed young man whose girlfriend has just dumped him? How many consultations had small crises embedded in them, such as pain over the liver in a woman who had had breast cancer two years ago? In how many were there reverberations of past crises? Maybe a teenager becoming a bit depressed brings back memories for the family of the suicide of his uncle. In how many might there be hidden crises? Take, for example, a fractured humerus (domestic violence?), recurrent indigestion (alcohol abuse?), recurrent urinary infections (sexual abuse?). In how many did it feel like a crisis for *you* but less for the patient: for example, when a patient presented with three problems in the last consultation of an already late surgery, or when you were trying to do a video surgery as a registrar and the sound on the video didn't work and you were already starting late? In how many consultations was the patient distressed but you remained calm and confident? Think of the 3-year-old boy who finds doing a poo terrifyingly painful and for whom each urge to go to the toilet is a major crisis.

Crises, little and large, are the 'driver' for much of our contact with patients. And these crises are rarely about one person only. At some level or other they involve other people and these are often, although, of course not always, members of the family.

Crises, of whatever shape or size – we are using the word broadly to capture many of the events, diseases, life changes, that occur in people's lives – affect individuals *and* families, the close ties, the contexts in which they live. As the reader will by now be aware, inside each person lies a whole family – revealed in the beliefs we hold about how to cope, the strategies we learnt from parents or other carers about what to do or not to do: stiff upper lip, talk to your mother, deny, ignore, bottle and splurge, adapt, panic.

Your crises

Imagine the crises that you yourself have had over the last week. They may be only small ones, like losing the keys to your car, or running late in a surgery, or feeling you were coming down with a cold. Jot them down.

Then think about how other people might have been involved in these 'crises'. What adjustments did others take or make? And how many of these were recurrent mini-crises with familiar dance steps?

What would have happened if you had not blamed your partner for mislaying the keys, or if you had not felt irritated with the receptionist for squeezing in two extras? Try to look at the interactive steps you and others took and ponder which, if any, you might change (or keep) if the crisis happens again.

Next please . . .

Mr F has his first unexpected coronary which happens suddenly without any prior warning signs. The whole family is temporarily destabilised. His wife is worried sick about his chances of survival and appears unable to attend to the normal household tasks. In addition she is full of self-blame as she cannot help connecting the coronary with a row that happened shortly before. Their 17-year-old daughter Jane feels not only sorry for her father but also for her mother, as she visibly does not cope. Mother in turn feels guilty for not being able to comfort her daughter sufficiently and this leaves the son Pete, aged 19, alone with his worries about his father's welfare.

Distressing though such a temporary disorganisation of family life is, given the circumstances, it is not abnormal. In a crisis situation the family's ordinary coping

Categories of crises

Different clinicians have been intrigued by different patterns of illness presentation and the ways in which people respond to these. They have developed some useful thoughts about how to be effective in varied circumstances. Here are a few references:

*   Chronic illness (Altschuler 1997)
*   Chronic pain (Mason 2003)
*   Bereavement (Fredman 1997)
*   Depression (Jones and Asen 2000)
*   Parasuicide (Asen 1998)
*   Domestic violence (Goldner *et al.* 1990)
*   Schizophrenia (Kuipers *et al.* 1992)

mechanisms may not be adequate to handle the new demands. The family's immediate response is influenced by how serious the family believes the illness is and how satisfied it is with the treatment and other support structures.

More please ...

A little time later son Pete steps temporarily into father's shoes and becomes the 'man of the house'. Mother has now taken on some of the responsibilities which had been allocated to her husband in the past. She is also considering doing some part-time work. Daughter Jane acts more independently and increasingly spends less and less time inside the home. When father is discharged home from hospital after about a month, he hardly recognises his family. He wonders whether there is still a place for him at home. His wife calls the GP and says that he is suffering from depression.

A template for thinking about families in crisis

There are lots of ways of thinking about families in crisis (Rolland 1987). How about this one? Draw a line across a page representing the individual or family's life cycle, thinking of all the transition points, including the genetic endowment and natural personalities of the individuals (Figure 11.1). This line represents the horizontal stressors of a normal family life cycle from birth to death. Above the line are the strengths, resources and resiliencies; below are the potential weaknesses and vulnerabilities. Threading across this line are the vertical stressors, which may be unexpected life events, cultural or religious beliefs, educational and employment issues. Also threading across the line are the family legacies of myths, beliefs and possibly secrets. Religious beliefs may hold a family together and appear above the line during bereavement but at a time of divorce may cause conflict. An unexpected pregnancy may pull a family together or make it fall apart. If the page of the family's life became a tapestry it would be an ever-changing one. The page can then be summed up by inviting the family or individual to make three headline statements about how the family works. These too can change with time.

Don't just think families – think context

Throughout this book we have written about the particular connections between people and their families. We have used a broad definition of family which includes those you were brought up with and those with whom you have a deep connection. But of course there will also be others, and not all of these are even human (never underestimate the importance of pets), with whom you interact closely and over long periods of time – the people who may become partners, the close friend, the mentor, the partner in the practice. There is very little in what we have written that cannot also refer to these other connections, 'partners in our dances', parts of our context: friends and enemies, colleagues, neighbours and others. So when thinking families also think 'context', asking what other relationships are important to this individual?

THE TAPESTRY OF FAMILY LIFE

Legacies	**Unexpected**	**Cultural**	**Education/Employment**
myths	illness/death	ethnic origin	financial
beliefs	pregnancy	religion	leisure
secrets			

Resiliencies
Resources

_____ **Family Life Cycle**

Vulnerabilities

Figure 11.1

This tapestry can be 'woven' or (more trendily put), 'co-constructed' by the clinician and family members. This is often an opportunity for the transfer of useful information. How often is it that professionals know risk factors but do not pass on the information to the family and its members in a way that could then empower them to take charge of the vulnerability and enable it to become a strength? For instance, the death of a parent of a young child is known to be a significant predictor for depression in later life. Discussing this early on with the family allows preventive measures to be put in place.

Next please ...

A middle-aged woman experiencing great difficulties with her teenage daughter traced the problems back to the death of her own mother when her daughter was 4 months old. She wished she had been able to talk through the loss at the time with a sympathetic professional, as she profoundly believed she would have bonded better with her daughter. Asked about her statements about her family she noticed that they had changed. 'We were a sad family for years but now we are stickers and survivors.' When drawing the diagram she talked about her past losses. This, she said, presented a vulnerability factor for the emotional health of her children. Discussing it with the health visitor, it struck her that this could be turned into a strength if she becomes appropriately protective of her children.

Next please ...

A woman abused by her uncle was helped, together with her husband, by her health visitor to reflect on how her own experiences could lead to a safer life for her baby daughter. This also helped the father to become centrally included in caring for his daughter and any future children. By drawing a diagram and seeing in a visual way her vulnerability gave her a determination

not to give herself the headline of 'Abused woman passes on trauma to her children'. She decided
she would rather have the headline of 'Determined woman with difficult childhood wins through'.

Next please . . .

Jack is a 3-year-old boy who has serious constipation. He has a new baby brother who makes
a lot of noise and hasn't smiled at him yet. He is sharing his mum, who had a caesarian
section and can't drive yet because of the operation. On the strengths side, he has a mum
who is sensitive to his needs and brought him speedily to the surgery, and a working dad who
is interested in what the primary care team says. He talks easily to the health visitor who
concludes that this family will negotiate their current crisis. However, the health visitor is also
concerned that mother might become postnatally depressed, given the family's rural isolation
and her operation. The family has plenty of resources – and also a health visitor who is
thinking preventatively. She asked mum: 'If Jack were to write a headline, what do you think
it should be?'

Next please . . .

At the other end of the life cycle we have Mr K, a retired engineer with bowel problems,
hypertension and a past history of a heart attack. Since his favourite granddaughter died of
a brain haemorrhage two years ago, he has not slept well and he is very 'nervy'. He rumi-
nates about his physical health endlessly and drives his devoted and devout Catholic wife to
distraction. He can't bear the effects of ageing and hates his poor mobility.

When Mr K's depression is treated with yet another antidepressant, how much
better do you predict he will be? How much do you think your assessment of his
likely improvement is affected by your own stage in the family life cycle and the
views you have about ageing? Do you see ageing as a crisis in itself or as a life
cycle stage? What could Mr K's headline have been? What will yours be when you
are 75?

In each of these four cases plotting the strengths and vulnerabilities onto the
template enabled the patient and involved family to see that they had vulnerabilities
– often events beyond their control: new baby, dead mother, dead granddaughter,
sexual abuse. These could simply be passively accepted or submitted to, but seeing
that there was another side of the line to move their vulnerabilities into strengths
allowed a reframing and the emergence of resilient coping strategies.

Family coping strategies

Families in crisis often seem to manage in ways that you may not understand and
sometimes in ways you would not choose. The routes by which patients navigate
their lives are wonderfully varied – that is partly what makes primary care such a
rich place to work. Systemic practitioners are interested in these routes and strategies. They are interested in the relationships families develop with the illnesses and
the crises they face. These could be termed coping strategies. We have already
talked about how depression can become another 'partner' in a couple relationship.

Just for a moment try thinking about depression, like other problems or illnesses, as a coping strategy. Does this frame allow different ideas to emerge about the apparent problem? Think about a family exhibiting extreme cheerfulness in the face of difficulty, or a couple who always ask you to make decisions and then are profoundly critical of you. They can be seen as families having coping strategies rather than just being reliable sources of intense irritation! Such feelings of discomfort may be an important clue that a particular coping strategy is in operation. It may feel a bit odd thinking about things that are commonly called illness and, by some, diseases – like depression or disordered eating, or chronic fatigue syndrome or irritable bowel syndrome or even aspects of asthma or chest pain – as coping strategies. And, of course, we take a Both/And position on this. These crises are behaviours *and* syndrome, *and* illnesses *and* problems *and* coping strategies *and* the hand of fate or God. Thinking about them as coping strategies can sometimes be more helpful than other ways of thinking about them both to the patient and to the family.

Understanding coping strategies

How do we begin to understand these coping strategies? The new baby arrives into a rich tapestry woven by the families of origin. The small infant has to make sense of his world and a huge amount of data in order to form relationships that will sustain him and hopefully help him thrive. The genetic endowment helps in this task and the capacity to learn from experience begins in the womb. He experiments and some of the feedback will be intrinsically more rewarding and apparently helpful – if only for short-term gains. This learning produces coping strategies, which the baby refines as time goes on. Over time the various developed coping strategies help him to manage anxiety and worry. Of course mum and dad – and significant others – also develop coping strategies that interweave.

Both/and positions

Over the years, systemic practitioners have made a journey from a binary choice 'either/or' stance to 'both/and' positions. It permits more than one perspective and view of any event – or behaviour – to be entertained at any one time. The dichotomy between self and system disappears in relational contexts. The 'both/and' position in this context can be traced back to Andersen (1987) with his depiction of dialogue and meta-dialogue in clinical work and Goldner (1992), describing the double perspective of feminism and systemic work with violence. This was heavily influenced by Bateson's concept of the 'double description' (Bateson 1972). He argued that obtaining more than one view of an event would help us to achieve 'binocular vision', gaining perspectives of both our observations and experiences (Jones 1993).

Those readers with a psychoanalytical bent may recognise in our descriptions of coping strategies some well-known 'defence mechanisms', such as projection, projective identification, denial, manic defence and displacement. We prefer to reframe these by using interactional and user-friendly descriptions.

Coping strategies

What follows in the main text is a set of coping strategies that individuals and families use in a whole variety of contexts and circumstances. None is specific to a particular crisis.

When you read through them we would encourage you to try to identify particular people or families where that particular coping strategy might be in use. Sometimes it will be an illness that triggers the strategy, sometimes some other life event. It is not, of course, an exclusive or exhaustive list.

This way of thinking is just another way of encouraging you to ask the question; 'What might be going on here?' And 'Is this way of framing the action helpful in moving forward?'

Playing the blame game – a way of coping with stress or anxiety

Next please . . .

Harriet is 16 and is part of a lively family, which often seems too expressive for everyone's comfort. She was brought to her GP by her parents, Mr and Mrs S, because of concerns about substance misuse. She looked sad and sullen. She said that when tensions are high she uses cannabis, which seriously worries her mother as her older brother had a drug problem. Mrs S then screams at her and it is only a matter of minutes before Mr S joins the fray. Both parents feel very strongly that there is something seriously wrong with their daughter, such as severe mental illness.

The Drama Triangle (Karpman *et al.* 1987) describes a triad consisting of *victim*, *rescuer* and *persecutor*. It can be represented in a diagram (Figure 11.2), which may help families to see in the form of a picture of how they might be functioning, and often reveals choices for them in how to behave. In the scenario above, Harriet could be described as the victim and mother as the persecutor. Mr S, when entering the scene, plays the role of Harriet's rescuer and he shouts at Mrs S, who then takes the victim position, with dad acting as the persecutor. Harriet re-enters the fray to rescue her mum by shouting at Mr S, who then becomes the victim and the shift of roles around the triangle is complete. When this diagram was drawn, the family rapidly worked out that this complete cycle could take less than five minutes, with everyone left feeling as though they had survived an eruption from Mount Etna.

This discussion was followed by a number of questions which each family member was asked:

- 'What are you worried about in this row?'
- 'What are you worried about in your own personal life?'
- 'What needs to happen to separate the two levels of worry?'

The conversation triggered by these questions resulted in:

- Mrs S wanting to find different ways of coping with her anxiety about Harriet's brother.
- Mr S wanting to find different ways of coping with his work pressures.
- Harriet wanting to find different ways of thinking and going about her transition to college.

When reflecting about these different anxieties, Mrs S commented that it was easier to focus just on Harriet than to think about her own worries. Mr S agreed that he had sleepless nights being anxious about his job (Figure 11.3).

This particular piece of family work with the three of them, over three 10-minute consultations, changed the focus and allowed each person to address their own anxieties. It probably could have been done with only two of them present or even one – by asking whoever was there to put themselves in the other people's shoes.

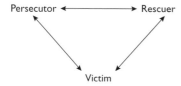

Figure 11.2

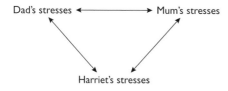

Figure 11.3

The Drama Triangle can equally be applied to difficulties with colleagues.

Next please ...

June, a health visitor, was concerned that a family she was involved with was being persecuted by social services and the court system. Each time she attended a case conference and mentioned this dynamic in as gentle a way as possible, she was rounded on and her sense of her own competence plummeted. The Afro-Caribbean mother of the family in question, Ms L, was living in an almost exclusively white northern town having moved from London. She was continually being told by her mother that she was no good as a mother. Her partner, who drifted in and out of the family home, would mount a staunch defence of her when he was in the family home, but she would then launch an attack on him in defence of her mother. It was at such times that domestic violence would occur. June had a good rapport with Ms L, which derived in part from the fact that she was very interested in comparing differing cultural parenting styles. She thought that Ms L was doubly disadvantaged by being black and having London ways. She also knew that Ms L's mother would often phone up the social worker and harangue her. In supervision one look at the Drama Triangle provided a new perspective. The placing of a label of victim, persecutor or rescuer on each of the players immediately invited new ideas about what was going on and how it changed at different stages of the dance. She shared her ideas with the social worker and then the mother. This improved working relations both professionally and within the family: everyone had descriptions for the different positions they assumed in quick succession.

Doing someone's dirty washing – or why do patients or clinicians accept all this unpleasant 'stuff' from others?

How often do you find yourself thinking 'She needs to let him stand on his own feet', 'She can't mother him for ever', 'That dad lets him get away with murder'. These are all part of the 'doing someone's dirty washing' coping strategy. The easiest visual description is that of the working of the amoeba, which can be adapted for use in the 10-minute consultation. An amoeba can be described as a single-celled organism which ingests and cleans up the environment around it. Some mothers – and very occasionally fathers – could be said to behave like amoebas, cleaning up the mess around their children, sometimes for much longer than is helpful for the child. They can also find it very difficult to let go. We find similar patterns in couple relationships.

Next please . . .

Mrs O is a 48-year-old woman with multiple sclerosis and severe bowel problems. Over the years the GP has got to know her story well. She is a great-grandmother because she had a daughter at 16, and so did her daughter and her daughter's daughter. She feels very guilty that she devoted so much time to her daughter that she forgot about her son who still lives at home. She still feels ashamed about the illegitimacy. She spends all her time when well running about after her family, giving them money, buying them presents. This all very well but her granddaughter is taking heroin and may lose custody of the baby. Her daughter has a drink and temper problem. Her husband threatens to leave unless he has a bit of time with her.

Her family life was drawn as a family of amoebae with her in the middle absorbing everyone's muddle and getting recurrently ill in the process. Everyone else was getting off scott-free and there wasn't room for her husband to have a relationship at all as she was so full of everyone else's dirty washing.

A solution diagram was then drawn with each individual carrying and taking responsibility for his or her own worries, emotional and financial. Mrs O could then see the possibility of a real relationship with her husband and more honest ones with her children and grandchildren. Looking at the solution diagram also enabled her to see how her major task was to learn to feel content when alone. Doing the dirty washing gave her a sense of closeness but one she was reluctant to give up. Finding new ways of being close took some time. She reported back in subsequent consultations about her amoeba family's closeness and distance. She also monitors her washerwoman status and has noticed a connection between relapses of her MS and taking on too much washing to do. The picture became a shorthand to describe instantly the pattern of family relationships.

This technique can also be used with families with adolescents who get into trouble with the law, including with parents of drug-addicted young people. These parents often pay court fines and plead that their child had extenuating circumstances (family tensions, loss of job, bereavement in the family) and you may find that you, the clinician, are doing the same! This is a classic example of doing the young person's dirty washing and not allowing them to grow up and accept full responsibility for their lives. 'Tough love' was what Haley (1979) called it. Seeing a visual representation of 'tough love' and the benefits for all helps families move through the life cycle stage of launching their children. One father of an anorexic girl used the 'dirty washing' metaphor quite literally. She had been spoilt by her anxious mother, who continually picked up her dirty clothes, washed and ironed them. They agreed that he could put any clothes left lying outside her room into a black bin liner. This was an important first step to enable her (and them) to grow up.

Using rose-tinted spectacles to look at silver linings while playing the glad game

Some people are born optimists; some people learn to be cheerful as a coping strategy that wins them friends. 'Laugh and the world laughs with you. Cry and you cry alone', as they say. Taken to its extreme, a persistent cheerfulness can be exasperating to live with, as sensible and necessary emotional discourse becomes unavailable within the family. As an optional coping strategy, flexibly used, it has its value and fun.

Next please . . .

Mr and Mrs D had been consulting their GP for support during their marriage breakup. The theme of the consultations had been to make a good job of this transition and to challenge the cultural assumption that all marriage breakup is necessarily bad and sad. One of the things about Mr D that had always irked his wife was his unbounded cheerfulness – she could never get him to listen when she felt sad. They decided to use his coping strategy to get them through the day of her moving out, which they had decided to do together. This worked well for them but was quite hard for their friends, who had offered to help, because they hadn't prepared them properly for cheerful banter at what is traditionally a sad event! It took some time before the friends joined in.

Next please . . .

Mr R's father had died when he was 10. His Christian family used cheerfulness as a coping strategy to manage this event. He did well and trained as a solicitor. When his wife died leaving him with three teenage children he continued to use this strategy and struggled to engage with the emotional consequences for his children. His two sons soon indulged in risky drug-taking behaviours and his daughter in risky sexual acting-out. The GP was unable to get him to look through anything other than rose-tinted spectacles as Mr R maintained: 'Well it's what all children do and I coped with the death of my father so they will cope with the death of their mother.' The GP asked Mr R to bring his three children into the surgery. It emerged that the Christian sense of smiling through life's vicissitudes, which had empowered him all his younger life, was a source of profound irritation for his children. Mr R had to learn other coping strategies to connect with his children's experiences.

What the eye doesn't see the heart doesn't grieve about – the use and abuse of denial

The phrase 'he's in denial' is commonly used to describe a reaction to trauma when someone is not taking in the full impact of something that has happened. It can be seen as an expected coping strategy after bereavement, as it has advantages of enabling people to organise funerals, get on with life until such time as they are ready to cope with more and more of the consequences of what has happened. Denial can be an 'integrity protector', stopping personal disintegration, and probably operates much of the time in most people when there are serious stressors. It becomes damaging at certain times such as when it contributes to domestic violence, sexual abuse, or acts of self-harm connected with alcohol problems and eating disorders. Hypothetical questions are helpful in this situation as they give a different dimension for the patient:

- 'Supposing you were able to remember how violent you were with your wife in the way the police describe, how would that feel different?'
- 'If you were your wife, what do you imagine it would feel like that she can remember every second of the violence and that you can remember none?'
- 'Supposing you began to be able to recall some of the violence, which bit do you think it would be easiest to remember?'
- 'If you could observe yourself when you were drunk, what would you see? What does it feel like describing another part of yourself you can't remember?'
- 'Drinking in some people distances them from the emotional consequences of their actions. If you hadn't been emotionally distanced in this way, how would you be acting differently now?'
- 'Supposing coming to terms with the consequences of alcohol/violence/sexual abuse takes time to work through, how long do you think it will take for you? What help do you think you will need to achieve this? What personal strengths and other resources do you have to enable this to happen?'

Black clouds, lead weights and treacle

Primary care practitioners have long been berated for 'missing depression' – and there are certainly examples of this. But we wonder whether clinicians operating in the complex space of primary care which spans lay and professional worlds have intuitively realised that it is not always useful to call these feelings and behaviours picked up by screening and diagnostic tools 'depression'. Depression can have some very useful functions and in these circumstances would benefit from renaming. Words that come to mind are: acceptance, sadness, anticipatory worry, willing submission, self-protection, avoidance, relationship glue, time for reflection. As a temporary strategy in the patient's repertoire it can be helpful and, on occasions, a wise decision to call the condition depression, but if it is out of control it can lead to loss of employment, loss of relationships, loss of physical health, death by suicide or physical disease. Questioning this is a delicate matter.

'It can sometimes be helpful in primary care to tell parents that they qualify for a diagnosis of 'adolescent parents' in that they have 'special needs' in this phase of the family life cycle. Adolescents can be extraordinarily demanding and parents often do not know where to turn for help.

Next please . . .

Mrs F is contemplating her children leaving home, needing HRT, waiting for a thyroidectomy and slowly coming off diazepam and refusing all offers of the GP's help.

- *'It seems to me that the sort of depressed way you are at present is very important and that to change things may bring up some issues which could feel unmanageable. It would help me to know what the disadvantages and advantages are to you of your present mood.'*
- *'Supposing you got better, how could you manage not to have extra demands put on you till you were ready? Who is the most important person to help you with this? Who is the least likely person to help you with this?'*

Next please . . .

Zamira, age 17, diagnosed with 'depression', said she did not want to get better because she did not want to grow up. Her GP changed the diagnosis to 'Peter Pan Problem' and put the following questions to her: 'Supposing you got better, how would you still be able to delay the business of growing up? Which bits of growing up would you like to delay? Which bits would you like to allow to happen? What would mum and dad say about this conversation? What was it like for mum and dad when they were your age?'

Next please . . .

Mrs A was the 'depressed' mother of teenage children who had noticed that the children are better behaved when she is going through a spell of low mood. This is what her GP asked her:

- *'When you are depressed your teenage children are more helpful around the house. What needs to happen to get them to be more helpful without you having to get depressed? Who can help you with this?'*
- *'Supposing you pretended to be depressed to get them to behave, how would you set about that? Who would you have to let in on the secret? Who would you exclude from the secret?'*

Depression and obesity are often linked. Another common factor in both treatment of resistant depression and treatment of resistant obesity is the presence of a partner who is critical and makes the patient feel put down. The 'resistance' can be seen differently in the light of the interaction. Partners of obese women often fear that their spouses will leave them if they lose weight and become more attractive to other men. They tend to make most of their critical remarks at mealtimes. This fear may often (but not always) be unfounded. Simple enquiry of this belief and questions around what happens at meals can make the issue clearer and help to maintain weight loss. Such questions have a routine place in diabetic, hypertension and coronary heart disease clinics, where family interventions are shown to improve outcome (McDaniel *et al*. 1990). Children are accurate observers in this situation. 'I don't understand dad when he says mum needs to lose weight 'cos he pours oil all over the food and gives mum massive helpings.' Clinicians can bring in the children virtually: 'If the children were here, what would they have to say about mealtimes?'

Similarly a less 'depressed' wife may be more likely to leave home. Discussion about this outcome may dispel fears or may raise important issues that are better addressed than repressed.

I won't let the b . . . d grind me down. Just get on with it

As primary care clinicians we do from time to time see resilient coping strategies in operation as families cope well despite extraordinary odds.

> ### Next please . . .
>
> *A 40-year-old psychiatric nurse was suffering from a manic state for the first time. He was determined to get through it without medication and persuaded his GP and psychiatrist that this was possible. He knew he had been stressed at work and his wife had not been able to help as her father had just died. He had had a childhood of profound neglect and felt that to go on medication would be to succumb to that. Over the next weeks he exercised, walked the fells and talked to his counsellor about learning to identify his vulnerabilities and triggers. Ten years on he is well and actively manages his mood as he is aware that mania is just around the corner if he is not vigilant.*

As clinicians we owe it to our patients to give them empowering resilient strategies in the face of potential enormous difficulty. Life is a challenge, not a steamroller!

> ### Next please . . .
>
> *Clare is 10 and has a long-standing relationship with the practice nurse, having attended the asthma clinic and talked about the difficulties of her parents separating two years ago. She is dyslexic. When she is brought by her mother to the GP with anal warts, the GP sends her to the practice nurse to ease the referral to social services for suspected sexual abuse. Clare said she wanted to see the nurse to tell her about the last bad day she had had with her Dad because he had called her bad names.*
>
> NURSE: 'When you decided to come and tell me about your dad calling you bad names, what did you want me to do about it?'
>
> CLARE: 'I wanted you to make sure I never go to Manchester again.'
>
> NURSE: 'That sounds as though you had a very difficult time. Sometimes when you have had a difficult time it helps to draw your family rather than talk about them. Would you like to do that?'

Whilst doing the drawing of granny who was 'fierce' Clare said that her dad had called her a bitch. The nurse explained that to help her get what she wanted – not to go to Manchester again – she would have to talk to her mum and asked if that was OK.

Clare's mum was shocked at the revelation of probable sexual abuse and said that her son was also edgy. However, she appeared to minimise the necessity of stopping trips. The practice nurse felt initially angry at this but regained her neutrality and became curious at this minimisation and what it signified. There were two possible reasons: one that the mother would have no help with the children, but more importantly that she was frightened of her ex-husband. The practice nurse encouraged her to voice what she wanted to happen and empowered her to phone social services herself straight away. The nurse phoned later to explain the careful work she had done. The nurse received several abusive phone calls from the father.

The practice nurse debriefed with the health visitor as the consultation had been draining. She saw in the records that there were many consultations for constipation and urinary infections. She wondered how the practice could have dealt with this earlier.

When the family gets into the body – thoughts about somatisation

Our language has a rich seam of mind–body metaphors: 'I've got you under my skin', 'I can't stand this', 'I can't swallow that', 'I can't stomach it'. The term 'somatisation' is a medical frame for patients presenting psychological problems through physical symptoms. It is as though the body copes with stress, which could seem intolerable if experienced directly in the mind. In this way somatising can be seen as another coping strategy.

Next please ...

Jo is 8 and has asthma. Whenever the practice nurse sees him with his parents they seem a loving family interested in his well-being, but she does notice that they sit on either side of him. Eventually she gets a story out of them that his first bad asthma attack occurred when they were having a row. His asthma settled as they stopped rowing and joined together to be worried about Jo. The nurse explained how tension can affect the smooth muscles lining the breathing tubes by direct effects of stress hormones, and by breathing too much and affecting carbon dioxide levels. She asked them if they were happy for Jo's asthma to be the regulator of their marital tensions. She then explained to Jo that his mum and dad would come and talk to her about their problems and thanked him for having brought them. She said he didn't need to carry on being poorly to get them sorted out.

Next please ...

Mrs C is in her late fifties and has a fat folder. She has had eight major bowel investigations over the last 15 years and consults very frequently for her irritable bowel syndrome. When her GP decided to take stock just before the ninth major investigation, she readily agreed to discuss her genogram. It emerged that her mother died of cancer when she had just given birth to her first child 'and you know that is when the pains began'. Four of her mother's siblings had died young of cancer; two of colonic cancer. She had one 80-year-old aunt alive. Her husband's side of the family had a similar sad tale. His twin brother had died of leukaemia and another brother in a road accident. Her husband had survived a serious myocardial infarction five years before 'and my goodness that brought the pain on'. Closer enquiry revealed that recently a close friend had died and her son had moved abroad. She had no difficulty making the link and was surprised that no one had asked her about her family history before. The gastroenterologist decided on planned reassessments of her colon and she decided she would rather come and talk about her feelings if the pain returned. Her consultation rate dropped. She remarked that it was as though her body had coped with the pain of losing her mother because she couldn't give in to it with the demands of caring for a small baby. Her mother had got into her body to be reawakened each time a real or threatened loss occurred. Interestingly, when her son was diagnosed with early bowel cancer her consultation rate didn't increase and she coped very well.

An anaesthetist and chronic pain specialist recently introduced to systemic ideas said: 'It's as though the family gets into the body – and what an uncomfortable place for a family to be – for the family and the patient.' How might it have been different for Mrs C if her GP had made the link earlier?

Painful stories

Chronic pain in its many forms is the mainstay of primary care, whether it is in the form of back pain, painful joints, rheumatoid arthritis or recurrent migraine. It is interesting to speculate on the reasons for this lest, as primary care clinicians, we go through the day with a biomedical lens that fails to see the patient's felt experience. Clinicians may feel that they need to ward off too many painful stories as a form of self-protection against burn-out, or they may believe that it is the doctor's role to diagnose and prescribe and the patient's role to get on with living with it. Doctors in particular have a belief that it is their job to make people better; patients who do not improve challenge this belief and can make the GP feel power-

The roar that lies the other side of silence

Not that this inward amazement of Dorothea's was anything very exceptional: many souls in their young nudity are tumbled out among incongruities and left to 'find their feet' among them, while their elders go about their business. Nor can I suppose that when Mrs. Casaubon is discovered in a fit of weeping six weeks after her wedding, the situation will be regarded as tragic. Some discouragement, some faintness of heart at the new real future which replaces the imaginary, is not unusual, and we do not expect people to be deeply moved by what is not unusual. That element of tragedy which lies in the very fact of frequency, has not yet wrought itself into the coarse emotion of mankind; and perhaps our frames could hardly bear much of it. If we had a keen vision and feeling of all ordinary human life, it would be like hearing the grass grow and the squirrels' heart beat, and we should die of that roar which lies on the other side of silence. As it is, the quickest of us walk about well wadded with stupidity.

George Eliot, **Middlemarch, Chapter 20** (Dorothea after her marriage and honeymoon with the dreadful Dr Casaubon)

less and redundant. Chronic pain comes with two major features in primary care: constant pain and pain of a relapsing sort with a spectrum of pain in between episodes. The patient and family with chronic pain may have a primary or a secondary relationship with the pain (Mason 2003). If they have a primary relationship then their lives revolve around the pain. If it is secondary, then the pain is part of what else they do in their day-to-day lives. Sometimes the nature of the pain may be such that despite individual and partner attempts to have a secondary relationship with it, the pain remains primary, in the foreground. However, there is a difference, Mason (2003) suggests, between an episode of pain being seen in the context of a secondary relationship with pain and with an episode of pain being seen in the context of a primary relationship with pain (after Pearce and Cronen 1980). Thus, it may sometimes be useful to ask questions of the patient and partner that address their relationship to these episodes.

Next please . . .

Clinician [to Mr M and his wife]: 'When these episodes are so painful that it is difficult to keep the pain in the background and it remains in the foreground, how do you both view these times?'

Mr M [in his mid-forties and a chronic pain sufferer]: 'Well sometimes I just say to myself I'm too tired to make an effort. I used to be bad at giving in to it but then I started to see it differently. Like, I see there's giving in in a bad way and giving in in a good way. I know that I try to fight the pain, not let it overtake me, so if I give into it sometimes I know it won't happen very often. That's giving in in a good way. But if I always gave in to it so that it sort of overtook me, that would be giving in in a bad way.'

Mrs M: 'He's right. He doesn't tend to give in to the pain so when he does I know it must be really bad. But if I thought he was giving in to it too much I would have a go at him because that would be no good for him or me. We'd end up arguing.'

Chronic pain is often structural, is ever present and has to be managed as part of the lived day. It has meaning for the patient and for each member of the family. If

Pain-full relationships (after Mason 2003)

1   A lack of fit between the patient's and significant others' beliefs concerning the management of the pain is likely to decrease or accentuate the difficulties in managing the pain.

2   Old (family of origin) and newer emerging scripts in coping with adversity, both for the person in pain and for significant others, is likely to aid or constrain the effective management of the pain.

3   Pain is a relational as well as an individual issue. Pain can best be managed by good teamwork and by being pro-active in engaging social support systems.

4   Uncertainty and concerns about the future and the condition exist both for the person with the pain and significant others. They need to be given a voice.

there is a primary relationship with the pain, then a family dance around the pain can develop which can make it seem as though the pain is unreal because it apparently serves a function for the family. Surgery and family can then get locked into an unhelpful and tiring way of relating, files get fatter and no one gets any relief.

Next please ...

Jo, 28, gets pain all the time in the skin of his upper body, which is worst over his head. He has had this continuously for eight years. He lives at home with his parents. Recently the pain was so bad he threatened to kill himself and was admitted to a psychiatric unit for a week, which he hated, in particular because they were unable to find any medication to numb the pain. He was a frequent attender. He had seen the community psychiatric nurse and been referred for brief psychotherapy to no avail. One of the GPs asked the practice nurse to meet with him and his family. They said that they would do anything to make the pain better and feel better as a family. The nurse said that she wasn't sure she could help the pain but that she might be able to help them as a family live with it better. She asked them if they wanted to try some family work and see whether it proved to be useful. Both parents and son agreed. Father attended frequently with work-related anxieties and chest pain. Mother was on antidepressants. The nurse decided to treat this information as confidential and to wait for the stories to emerge as she had never met any of the family. She wondered why Jo hadn't left home.

To help her get her head around the family they agreed to do a genogram. Dad was an only child, his mother had had a stillborn child before him. She was a bossy woman who controlled everything he did until her death 10 years before, a year after her husband's death. Jo's dad became visibly tearful at this point. He became quite engaged thinking about how the stillbirth could have affected her relationship with him and made it difficult to let him go when it came for time to leave home. Jo's mum described her own family as not being very close and spoke about a sense of not knowing what was in her life for her when her son left home. She looked very sad. Jo said that actually he had always felt his grandparents were his real parents and that he had felt so sad when they died but that no one had noticed, not even when his dog had also died. He thought his dad had started drinking at this point. The nurse fed back that they had had some sad events in their lives that had shaped how people could and couldn't leave home. Somehow the sad events had stopped people thinking they could have a future or even enjoy life in the present.

The second consultation involved mother and son. They reported that dad was a different man, having made some sense of his life and was being more thoughtful with his son. Further detail of the drinking and fear of violence emerged. The drinking had stopped as a result of Jo's admission to hospital – dad feeling it was all his fault. Mum admitted to her recurrent depression, which surprised her son until he related how he had kept his pain a secret for four years. He told her she needed to 'get a life' and reminded her of things she used to do. He decided not to come to the next session as 'Mum needs the help now'. Over the next few consultations Jo's mum was helped to take charge of her life again and to look at ways the changes the family had made could be consolidated so that it was impossible to slip back. Jo reported that family life was completely different but that the nurse had been right that the pain was no better at all. Family life being better did, however, help him to live with his pain.

While reflecting on this case in supervision the nurse said that she had felt very disappointed that the pain was no better because she was so sure she had identified the psychosocial antecedents to the pain with the loss of grandparents and dog. This was doubly challenging to her because as a nurse she had wanted to make his pain better and she had had a deep conviction that it was all psychological. Some time was spent wondering about the experience of a patient encountering professionals who hold deep-seated beliefs in their magical powers and fixed ideas about the causes of symptoms. In the course of five consultations, lasting 30 minutes each, they moved from having a primary relationship to the pain as a family to a secondary one.

I can't swallow this, it sticks in my throat – eating disorders and coping

Next please . . .

Sarah became anorexic at the age of 15. She could remember the moment when she stopped eating properly. She was sitting on a bus going to school feeling anxious because she had to give a presentation that day to her class. She felt a tightness in her chest and thought she wouldn't be able to swallow anything. She stopped eating and rapidly started to feel confident in managing not to eat. Her GP asked her: 'Supposing someone had explained to you that day about how adrenaline and anxiety make people's gullets go into spasm. What might have happened differently?' She looked wistful and said it would all have been a lot less complicated if she'd understood better how her body worked.

Eating disorders could be described – or constructed – as another variety of somatisation disorder. In the beginning they may arise out of family distress and perhaps mistaken understandings of how the body works.

In both these cases a worry had got into the body. Patients and families like to know how their bodies work, as in Sarah's case. They like to know about the effects of adrenaline and hyperventilation on smooth muscles. They are intrigued to learn about adrenaline and how it produces flight, fight or fright reactions. They know what they are managing if they know the detail and they can feel a great sense of achievement in controlling their bodies and lives. Many of the difficulties would not be so great, perhaps, if they were explained in detail earlier, and crises could be averted as was undoubtedly the case with Jane.

Primary care clinicians can make a great deal of difference in this area. Like any other area of difficulty, problems with eating do not start as full-blown anorexia or

Coping strategies

This is an exercise that proves useful if carried out in a workshop setting.

Choose a coping strategy – as described in this chapter. In groups of four or five create a family with a primary care team professional. Choose a stress – bereavement, onset of diabetes, drug or alcohol problem. Have a five-minute conversation about this stress, using just one chosen coping strategy to discuss what the family will do next. Stop and reflect on the positive and negative aspects of talking in this way. Repeat the same, this time using a different coping strategy. Repeat with family members using different coping strategies. Try to create a 'dirty washing' scenario with a mother looking after everyone's emotional needs.

bulimia. They have to start at the beginning with some change in the way a person relates to eating or to weight or to body image. The pathophysiological changes and ingrained family and personal behavioural patterns so often talked about as the characteristics of anorexia or bulimia are often not seen early on when new steps may have been tried, but are not 'fixed' or predictable. At this early stage a timely intervention with a systemic lens can be extremely useful.

Next please ...

Jane (16) was brought to her GP by her mother because her periods had stopped for three months and she had lost a lot of weight. The surgery knew the family well as all three daughters and mother were frequent attenders. The dad was registered with a different practice. The possibility of pregnancy was vehemently denied and there seemed no evidence of hormonal problems. The GP decided to be brave and invited the whole family to attend for an hour. She explained this to her sceptical partners as being about 10 minutes for each family member, which was nothing out of the ordinary for that family in one week.

The family session needed little input from the GP, as the father eventually said he knew why they were there. It was because Jane was feeling stressed because she slept in the next bedroom to her sister and her sister's boyfriend and couldn't help hearing them at night. Jane knew that her parents disapproved. Subsequent to the session, Jane's sister moved out and into her own flat. Jane then started eating again, her periods returned and 18 months later was back asking to be put on the pill. The consultation rates for all four women dropped over this time.

The issue of permission

Throughout this book we have been encouraging you to explore beyond the symptom and beyond the individual, to set the story in context and to be curious and enquiring of the context. It is important to seek permission for this, to have explanations for why you might want to ask about other aspects of the story. 'It would help me a great deal in understanding what you are going through to know a little about who is around to support you?' 'Would you mind if I asked a little more about how other people in your family think about your problem?' Or using the symptom as a route to the context: 'When you first started to get angina, what did your partner do? And now that you have been getting the pain for three years?'

This issue of permission is a tricky one. If people have not made the connections themselves they may be puzzled by your interest in exploring the context. However, it is usually quite easy to explain where you are going and you will often discover that people are much more 'tuned in' to the connections than you are. Nevertheless, be careful that you do have permission and watch for any clues that you may be nearing the limit of the permissible territory (Zigmond 1978).

Many people are happy and able to manage their crises themselves. But there are circumstances where it pays to at least think about being more actively involved:

- Acute major crises
- Heart attacks
- Severe or life-threatening illnesses.

Circumstances where it appears that adaptation and coping may be going awry may include:

- Unexpected length of illness or lack of expected recovery
- Unusual levels of engagement or disengagement by other family members
- Psychosomatic symptoms in spouse or sibling
- Non-compliance with medical regimen
- Intense feelings of guilt, anger, despair and worry
- Avoidance of talking about illness/denial/secrecy.

Coping strategies and clinicians – burnt out or fired up?

It is not only families but also clinicians who use coping strategies. Some of these are our own and some are induced by the demands of the patient and family. Our patients expect a varied range of responses from us.

This GP remembered the emerging evidence base for different personality structures and cancer survival, but she could not think of a way to introduce these ideas tactfully. Maybe these questions could have helped:

- 'Supposing you both became very positive about this cancer and your chances and that you forgot to think about it so much, would that have any benefits for you?'
- 'Sometimes we seem to have quite depressing conversations about your cancer. Supposing one day I had received an optimistic report from the oncologist and was very upbeat with you, what would that be like for you?'
- 'Supposing one of you decided before the other to take a positive stance about all this, what would it be like having two different views in your house? What might other members of the family say?'

Next please ...

Two women going for breast surgery for malignancy had very different requirements of the professionals they encountered. One wanted an optimistic approach with only just as much detail as she herself asked for. She said that she and her husband couldn't cope with it any differently, because she had only just moved to the area and she had quite enough else to cope with as the children were settling into new schools. This request was quite difficult for the GP, who felt very sorry for the patient having to cope with so many simultaneous demands. She also felt uncomfortably edgy, having to talk over-optimistically to the patient. She wondered what it was like for the children in this family and asked some questions over subsequent consultations:

- *'How will you know when it may be time to have a different way of coping with this?'*
- *'How would you know that the children are not affected differently from you? Who might be the best person for them to talk to? You, your husband, teachers, friends, other family members?'*

The other patient was quiet and meticulous. She wanted to be involved in all the thoughts and decisions with her equally sombre husband. The GP found she felt quite depressed talking to this woman and started worrying about this ponderous approach allowing the cancer cells to invade the woman's body. (You see, doctors are just as influenced by their own ideas as by those of the patient!) She found herself thinking about how different patients' immune systems are affected by their attitudes.

Teams now divide up the work when dealing with emotional illness: community psychiatric nurses, counsellors and psychologists now all work in primary care and have specialist sessions that help to spread the load. This way of working may have an advantage in diminishing the stress of listening to distress, but it may have the disadvantage of dissociating the clinician from the patient's emotional journey. Unless constructively and responsibly managed, enabling the clinician to continue working and to refer or collaborate with other professionals with specialist skills, this dissociative process can reduce the primary care team's 'immune system', allowing stress to infect the team spirit. At worst it can lead to poor patient care and also to burn-out in the clinicians.

Sharing the load

Think about your health centre.

- What three statements might the practice make about its approach to work?
- Which coping strategies does it use as a whole team to manage the stress of the work? Who is most likely to get depressed?
- Who manages work with cheerfulness?
- Which staff go off sick with bodily pains?
- Who in the practice resorts to alcohol?
- Who in the practice pretends that things are fine when others say they aren't?
- Who in the practice does others' dirty washing?
- How flexible are all these coping strategies both individual and group?
- How often are there victims, perpetrators and rescuers around?

Roots, trunk, shoots, fruits and seeds

Putting it all together

> This chapter covers:
> O   The toolbox of ideas for changing your own practice
> O   How to sow seeds in the whole primary health care team
> O   The importance of developing the organisation as well as your self
> O   Working across organisations
> O   One hundred and one uses for a systemic practitioner in primary care!
> O   (Not much really!)

Making it happen in practice – a toolbox of ideas

We hope you reach this chapter fired up with enthusiasm for the way of thinking and consulting that we are proposing. Your enthusiasm will take you a long way in actually achieving change in the way you and your practice works. It strikes us that simply being still 'alive' to the richness of the consultation is often the critical factor. In some ways it does not matter which theory or technique is currently interesting you – neurolinguistic programming, cognitive behavioural therapy, solution-focused therapy, patient-centred consulting or systemic practice – it is the fact that you are still interested that counts! We know from extensive research and from different perspectives that what counts most is thoughtful, listening and respectful consultations with the people you see (Silverman *et al.* 1998). If this book has simply helped you 'stay alive', 'curious' and thoughtful in your encounters with patients we have achieved something.

Systemic practice makes a difference

Nevertheless, we also think that the particular ideas and ways of working that we talk about have importance both for you and for your patients. We are keen that you not only find them interesting, but also find ways of making them an everyday part of your practice. And changing your consulting style is much harder.

You are all extremely busy. Those in work in the twenty-first century, particularly in Europe and the USA, but perhaps elsewhere as well, are working harder and longer hours than ever before. And this is certainly true in health care and in primary care. Not only is primary care still rightly designed, in the UK at least, to offer a universal open access and therefore essentially reactive work setting, but we are also being encouraged to design for proactive, population-based care, as well as taking centre stage, albeit with other agency partners, in designing and commissioning services. The tasks that fall to the primary care team and its members bear only passing resemblance to those that faced the oldest author of this book when he first entered practice in the 1950s!

However, the central tasks of seeing, listening, being with and doing to patients and their families are the same. So how, when there is so much to do, can we learn to do anything differently? It is certainly a challenge and there is no doubt that it will take time – time enough to read this book, time enough to think and time enough to practise something different and reflect on the results. That sounds like a lot of time but the great news is that we already practise seeing patients perhaps 20 to 40 times each day. So it is possible to practise small steps repeatedly until we change the default mode of practice and the new behaviour becomes embedded.

Changing the way you work

Perhaps the first step is being aware of what you currently do, actually taking the time to think about how you behave when seeing patients right now. In particular, notice how you behave when you are under pressure, running late, on a Friday afternoon, when you know you have a meeting to go to – the default mode of practice. It is then that you recognise the deeply ingrained behaviours you learned earlier – from your family of origin, from your culture, school and perhaps most significantly from the way you were trained. Much of this training was set in specialist settings with individual patients 'extracted' from the fabric of their lives, seen in crisis and under pressure.

The default mode, or what the North Americans call 'working at muscle memory level' – where there is little conscious interference between perception and consequent behaviour – usually has plenty of linear causality in its thinking, often ignoring details that do not fit, wrestling people's stories into preformed explanatory models and diagnostic categories. The default mode is selective in its curiosity, and inquisitiveness, with a ready-made set of hypotheses. Default modes jump from problem to solution with ease. They are crucially important because much of our work has to go on at this level. It probably saves our lives as practitioners and at times certainly saves patients' lives. But it can also constrain us and certainly makes new learning harder.

The more experienced clinicians will have already done much work in adjusting and monitoring their default mode settings. For instance, you may have learnt to wait longer before interrupting a patient at the start of a consultation. The average time in one North American study was 18 seconds from the start of a patient's story to first interruption by clinician. Most patients will take under two minutes to finish if allowed to (and usually reveal both reasons for attending and often the solution to their difficulties within that time). Many British practitioners will have ICE, the Royal College of General Practitioners mantra – eliciting the patient's Ideas, Concerns and Expectations – as a default mode setting.

Different professional groups have different default modes and often do not realise that theirs is unique to them. Much interprofessional relationship difficulty lies in not making overt these particular ways of thinking and working.

How can we embed a new way of thinking and doing into the default mode and how can we pull out of the hat different ways of working that suit a particular

Default mode settings

Have some fun either on your own or at the next practice meeting or learning event: identify your own default mode characteristics and have a guess at those of other team members.

One way of helping you to identify your default mode settings is to attempt to keep a bit of your brain/consciousness/sense outside or 'meta' to the consultation. This is an art or skill that needs to be learnt. It is similar to thinking about process rather than content (Neighbour 1987).

situation? We hope that the sequence of ideas and skills put forward in this book will help in developing yourself as a systemic clinician. You have already started showing an interest in developing your communication skills by picking up this book. What about making a bit of a commitment to the ideas? Perhaps you could ensure that it is discussed in your appraisal and in your personal development or PREP plan, lest it become an undercover and subsequently undermined secret! Then there is a forum for deciding what you wish to achieve over the next year and a forum for feeding back the results.

Solution-focused trained clinicians might write a letter to themselves beginning: 'In a year's time, when I award myself an A for improving my systemic skills I will have achieved . . .' (put at least three things you will do). Remember your A grade is about improving your practice, not about measuring up to some unachievable gold standard practised by the most experienced family therapists in the country (Zander and Zander 2000)!

Working on the family of origin (FOO)

Doing your own genogram will show you patterns that you may be able to recognise in the families you like or find a challenge. You will be clearer about 'trigger families' or people who 'press your buttons', who might upset you or make you behave in ways that are not characteristic (Hardy and Laszloffy 1995). Working on your own family of origin issues either on your own, with a trusted colleague or in formal supervision can be a very useful way of examining some of the unspoken threads of belief and behaviours that you bring with you into the consulting room. Primary care clinicians are perhaps unique in doing enormous amounts of mental health 'work' in their professional lives with almost no supervision or external support. Working on 'FOO' can be a start.

Working out the life cycle issues you and your family are going through may help explain why teenage patients are often at your door, or older women ask if you are going to be one of those lady doctors who stay in the practice, or you find yourself quizzing your patients about the best way to cope with the ageing process! 'Physician heal thyself' comes to mind!

Having practised on yourself, you then may find yourself having life cycle conversations with the practice nurse about your teenage children, or broken nights or poorly parents, and in your mind you construct genograms whenever you 'talk family'. This all then leads to doing a genogram with a patient, stumbling at first, but gaining in confidence as you do more. Some time later doing genograms may start to become embedded in your 'muscle memory' and you have begun the process of 'never being the same again'. Systemic ideas are transformational.

You may find that as you start to ask more questions about life cycle transitional tasks and patients start to give you feedback such as 'You really have got the point quickly, doctor' or 'You know what you're talking about don't you, nurse?' That sort of feedback encourages further adventures into the next stage of asking more interesting questions. To do this successfully is more of a challenge and takes some discipline as tired default mode readily goes back to medical questions. The number of potential questions we have presented you with in this book is, we suspect, at times overwhelming, so the task needs to be broken down into manageable chunks. Take a list of three questions you could easily ask most of your patients and put them on your desk. Over a couple of days ask most patients, for instance, about what other family members have to say about their illness, whether it is a cough or a cancer. One practice nurse was very open about the fact that she kept her book of circular questions in her drawer. She would say to patients: 'I have a book of wonderful questions in my drawer. I'm just going to have a look and see if there is just the right question to ask you now to help us move things on a bit.' We know this sounds wacky, but patients are extraordinarily tolerant of professionals – they really want you to keep thinking and learning, and they can recognise a better outcome when they see one!

Having got more confident in asking more interesting questions you will then notice that there is frequently more than one person in the room. Choose just one question you can ask whenever this happens. And then see what happens. If it helps make a shift, then it is more likely that you will use it again.

The importance of the feedback loop

It is the feedback loop that seems to be the most important thing of all. If, as a GP, you refer someone for a second opinion but do not hear any feedback about it for six months, the chance of you learning much from the exercise is limited. If, on the other hand, you have a conversation with the specialist the next day you may never need to refer someone with that query again – you will have learnt! It is no different with the ideas in this book. Keep them in your head and they will never change what you do; practise them and there is a chance! Listen to the feedback and respond to it and there is then even more of a chance.

This is why, throughout the book we have offered you 'Fruits' – lists and take-home skills – to act as *aides-mémoire* on your desk, and 'Seeds' – suggestions for exercises and tasks for you to try out in real practice. There is no way the germination rate will be 100 per cent, you may only try one in two of the seeds and find only half of them useful, but if you do not attempt to grow any of them you are unlikely to change your default mode settings very much!

So far but no further?

At this point you may find that you plateau out. It seems you have got the gist, tried one or two things, had a few successes but find that you often default to 'old mode'. It works OK but you wish you could get a few more of those questions under your belt, generate more imaginative hypotheses, get one or two more people into the room.

Now is the time when it would be helpful to have a 'buddy' with whom you can talk your experiments over. Your buddy does not need to be someone who has been on a formal family therapy training course, he or she can be simply someone who is interested in families and improving their own professional practice. Often a practice-based mental health worker fulfils this role well. Your buddy may be interested to work alongside you and get caught up with the curiosity that drives the whole of systemic thinking. This is the beginning of forming a collaborative relationship. These collaborative relationships across and within organisations are what underpin the success of systemic work. Through your relationship with your buddy you learn about the most important things to communicate and to question.

Changing your relationship to your team

By forming a collaborative relationship you have stepped out with your growing toolbox into the team. What will the rest of the team make of it? Will they see you and your buddy as having a good alliance or will they feel threatened? Will they see you as a new dumping ground for the problems they don't want to see? Whatever happens, a team dance begins and can be capitalised on.

Before becoming an evangelist for your newly formed but still vulnerable ideas and skills, it is a good idea to take stock. What do you know about this team of yours? What do you know of its history and development? What do they all know of each other? It is best not to make assumptions.

Understanding who you work with

How many of us go into a new job, one which consumes half (if not more) of our waking day and earns us the money we need to keep us alive, not knowing the history we are stepping into? If work were considered to be a marriage, how differently would you enter into it?

Collaboration in primary care

Much has been written about collaboration in primary care, particularly between generalists and mental health specialists (Seaburn *et al.* 1996, Cummings *et al.* 1997, Blount 1998). Most of this literature comes from North America, where educational and delivery systems split 'mental' and 'physical' more surely than almost any others in the world. Therefore those pioneers attempting to heal the split have been doing an exciting and creative job, with a whole organisation devoted to improving collaboration – the Collaborative Family Health Care Coalition (http://www.CFHA.net).

We would love to tell you more about this area of practice but suffice it to say that there is a great deal of difference between a mental health worker using a room in your building – what might be called 'co-location' or 'shifted outpatients', and a mental health worker and you working together, using corridor consultation, joint work, case discussion and the same coffee cup.

The empire of primary care has been growing despite initial fears of attached staff eroding the territory of the GP. A practice may be visited by consultants, psychologists, chiropodists, speech therapists, to name but a few. The development of the role of the practice manager has coincided with a profound shift in the sense that the GP is the king of the primary care castle. This also occurs at a time when nursing is espousing the demands of rigorous protocol-organised delivery of services, for instance, with diabetes, asthma and, in some areas, depression clinics. Practice managers (PMs) are increasingly behaving as managing directors, GPs as company directors and some PMs are profit-sharing partners.

These changes are fundamental to supporting the role of GPs as general physicians, general psychiatrists and minor op surgeons, with nurses stepping in to fill the breach of triage for minor and self-limiting illnesses and doing much of the work of child health clinics and contraception. These changes also create powerful dynamics that can silence the small systemic voice if ignored but can satisfyingly amplify the systemic voice if espoused. How to go about it?

The British health system in 'middle age'

Let us apply some life cycle theory to primary health care. Think about what you know and don't know of your health care system locally and nationally, its history, hierarchy and power struggles.

Birth
The National Health Service was 'born' in 1948 and a year later 80 per cent of GPs were working single-handed, mainly helped out by their wives who were often nurses.

The family starts to come together
In the 1960s the new contract revolutionised practices and the emphasis was on attaching health visitors and district nurses employed by the Health Authorities (HAs). In 1970 75 per cent of health visitors and 68 per cent of district nurses were attached. In the 1970s and 1980s the role of practice nurse was developed – from 1500 in 1977 to 18,000 in 1991.

New members keep getting added to the family of general practice
In 1972 Patient Participation groups were formed. In 1980 only six districts did not have a community psychiatric nurse service. By 1989 80 per cent of GPs worked in group practices, with the tendency being to larger and larger groups.

The power of some members may be waning slightly
The 1990s was the decade of the practice manager and also saw an explosion of provision of counselling into primary care.

The primary care family motto/guiding belief may also be changing
The twenty-first century has seen the development of proactive care for those with long-term physical and mental health problems. The rise to potential power of primary care organisations, the electronic record and a myriad other developments, including an increasing number of central targets.

Suppose you decided to take on the role of anthropologist to the team and ask questions about their professional histories and the changes they have seen. Having gained all this information, imagine a sculpt of the primary health care team. A sculpt is a freeze frame view of a team at a point in time. For a sculpt to fit with life cycle ideas, you can have one end of a room representing the past and the opposite end representing the future, with the positions of the professionals determined by the length of time they have been with the practice and with each professional looking towards past, present or future. Such a sculpt could be done with a systemic facilitator at an away day. It is a potent way for people within a team to understand their position within that team. If you were to draw maps of the relationships of the staff within primary care and their relationships to other organisations and agencies, how would they have changed over the period 1950 to 2010? How might they change in the future? You could also do a genogram of your primary health care team or the family circles – even attempt some amoeba drawings. All these techniques can be used to explore hierarchies and team relationships.

Next please . . .

A psychologist was asked to help a three-partner practice with some team building. The psychologist had known the practice for two years, had been helpful with the patients and was seen as someone who offered a variety of differing ways of working with the practice. She decided to do a modified version of a Family Circles Method with the team. The practice had undergone several changes, with a receptionist being promoted to practice manager in the previous year and each member of staff had difficulty defining where they stood in the pecking order as a result of this change. One of the partners had wanted someone from outside the practice with business experience to be appointed instead. He positioned the practice manager beneath him in the hierarchy whereas the other two partners saw her as alongside them. The nurses saw themselves lower in the order of things and still seemed to feel they were there to do what the doctor asked them to do. It seemed this balance would change when the primary care team took over the management of the practice nurses. Interesting questions were asked:

- *'Supposing in five years' time the practice manager was at the top of the hierarchy and both doctors and nurses were her employees, what would the advantages and disadvantages of that be?'*
- *'If that were the case would it be more or less easy for the doctors and nurses to get on as equals?'*

These and other questions made some of the dynamics more overt, encouraging more open discussion.

Another interesting game for an away day or even a lunch-time meeting is called 'Job Descriptions'. This appears very basic, but having heard an experienced GP saying at a conference that she could not role play a health visitor because she did not know what a health visitor did, we certainly feel it has a value! With rapidly changing roles, professionals may need to be reintroduced to each other from time to time. With the speed of the primary care day, sometimes even introductions never happen! Use a flipchart with a job title on each piece of paper (GP, practice nurse, practice manager, health visitor, counsellor, psychologist, district nurse, receptionist, secretary, dispenser) and ask participants to write a job description and a description of what training they thought people had had. Each person writes a sentence on each flipchart page except that referring to their own job. (Flippant remarks are allowed!) The holder of the job then has to read out their job description and comment on what is wrong and what is missing. They can also be invited to talk about their hopes for the future. In one practice the person most affected by this game was the counsellor, who having attended the practice for several years had not felt part of the team until that day. The staff were interested in the varied counselling trainings she had done and became curious as to what referrals she liked to see best. In another practice the whole team had their misperceptions about all community psychiatric nurses having a general nursing training informed. The game also opens the way for discussion about nurses feeling put upon by GPs wanting urgent ECGs and blood tests. Staff often do not know of each other's past interests and skills.

Change in you, change in the organisation

Your behaviour and ability to practise in new ways is not only related to the effort you put into learning new skills. Nor is it only related to better understanding the team with whom you are working. It is also closely related to the organisational structure and function of the place in which you work. Changing the way you work often needs changes in the way the organisation behaves or is designed.

Next please ...

One of the authors had been going on for years about the importance of offering patient infor- mation leaflets to patients during his consultations. He knew the evidence base, showing that patients often complain about a lack of information, that they only take in 30 per cent of what the clinician says, that information often helps grow a sense of agency which is directly related to better mental health. And yet he noticed that he still didn't give out information as often as he could have done. He took a moment to reflect and realised that one of the constraints was the time it took for his printer to print out the leaflet. When the patient and he arrived at the point in the consultation when a leaflet was thought to be a good idea it was usually within a minute of the end of the time. The printer took two minutes to print two pages. Solution – change the printer for a faster, laser printer! Leaflet distribution went up 10 times!

Similarly when the practice decided as a whole to adopt a set of mental health leaflets and start using them with patients as a way of helping clients help themselves, the difficulty was not in getting everyone to sign up to the idea, it was making it happen. There are many steps between having the leaflets somewhere in the building and having the right leaflet in the right patient's hand with the right advice and follow-up. This requires a number of organisational changes – leaflets in each room, someone tasked to replenish them, a teaching session on the content of the leaflets, and a macro on the computer to improve recording of the new activity so we can see whether it really is happening.

It is worthwhile thinking through what changes in the organisation may help you change and sustain change in your own behaviour.

Involving other systemic practitioners

At this point your systemic surgery is getting complex! Maybe you are thinking of holding a family clinic, maybe you identify more complex problems and want to

Miracle seeds working on the organisational system

Supposing you were to convert your entire surgery's working day to being completely 'family sensitive', what would be different?

- Genograms would be standard and with the appropriate software on the computer to draw them or to scan in the messy useful ones that everyone draws!
- You would have in the waiting room the invitation to family members to attend and reception staff would be clued up for this to be a good idea.
- You would have family record cards.
- Issues of confidentiality would be clear within the team.
- A health visitor and a GP would have had an introductory systemic training – perhaps consisting of 10 two-hour sessions at fortnightly intervals. These two would have enthused others to join them in collaborative working. Other members of the team would have attended 'family sensitive' training, to raise awareness. All team members should be able to work out life cycle stages and have a basic knowledge of the PPRACTICE assessment.
- You might be thinking of having a specialist family clinic (though by now each surgery will seem like a family clinic!).

work with them yourself. Finding a systemic supervisor could be helpful. There are many ways in which this could work:

- Whole team case discussion
- Individual supervision
- Supervision of the most interested clinicians
- Supervision of doctors or nurses in their own professional groups
- Live supervision/collaboration during ordinary surgery time
- Collaboration in surgery with specially selected patients
- Consultation to network meetings/child protection core groups
- Consultation to training especially around mental health topics or adaptation to chronic illness.

Systemic supervision in primary care does not have to be one hour for one family! Useful work can be done with 10 minutes for each family, thereby covering six families in one hour (with perhaps a 'double appointment' for a slightly more tricky one).

Next please . . .

A systemically trained practice nurse was aware that members of a family under her care were collecting professionals like bees to honey. The father had a drug problem relating to post-traumatic stress disorder following a time in the army in Bosnia. He was seeing a drug and alcohol worker and awaiting referral for EMDR (eye movement desensitisation and repro-cessing). The mother was depressed and pregnant so was seeing GP, health visitor, midwife and community psychiatric nurse (CPN) (who thought a referral to psychology would be a good idea). The daughter was 'hearing voices' and had a CPN from the Children and Adolescent Mental Health Service (CAMHS) team, who was muttering about child protection issues. The family were frequent attenders, often making appointments with the nurse to talk about all that was going on in their lives as well as appointments with the three partners. In supervision it seemed a network meeting of professionals would be a good idea. The meeting created a clearer structure for working with a minimum sufficient network, with the psychologist doing couple work to look at the impact of family of origin legacies on the current way of relating as a couple and with a professional network. She would liaise with the practice nurse, whose brief was to organise the primary health care team so that only the nurse and one doctor gave appointments to the family. The health visitor and CPN from CAMHS were to work in partnership. The drug and alcohol worker was not needed. The midwife's role was defined as being strictly antenatal care with any psychological worries being fed back to the health visitor.

Next please . . .

A five-partner practice requested systemic facilitation to discuss a demanding case with the whole team. The woman was a frequent attender at the surgery and a major user of out-of-hours services. She was pregnant, her children were on the at-risk register and her husband was due to appear in court for assault. Many potent and relevant issues were raised about the safety of staff, confidentiality and the structuring of the professional network.

The primary care team had not yet adopted a policy on the management of aggressive patients and as an issue in a rural area it had not been raised significantly amongst the health visitor group, who had only recently had a team leader created. The health visitor had thought she was a 'wimp' for being frightened to go to the house on her own. The social worker explained the policy of his organisation with its clearer distinctions about staff safety. Both CPN and midwife volunteered to accompany the health visitor in future. It was thought that if there was that degree of concern expressed by an experienced practitioner, perhaps the children were not safe at home at all.

The changing nature of the team outlined above means that belief systems about issues such as confidentiality need revisiting, establishing and documenting. The 'pretending not to know' of receptionists masquerading as confidential practice could be seen as quite dangerous where risk is involved and a practice may struggle to contain difficult patients by creating rules for receptionists, such as allowing patients to see only one doctor, making timed phone calls, etc. The practice manager was worried about the stress created amongst her receptionists by this case.

The core group restructured its authority, with the CPN being seen as the key worker for the time being. Any changes of psychotropic medication by GP or psychiatrist were to be discussed with him as he had the knowledge of the ups and downs of working with someone with a borderline personality disorder. This was seen as an important dynamic as it would then give the patient a sense of a team working together. The midwife was to join the group as she had seen the mother through all her previous three pregnancies. This challenged the view of the midwife as being a weighing and measuring person of limited availability. She also knew the pregnancy history of other members of the family and as such was a useful source of helpful professional gossip.

The practice covered all these issues in 40 minutes!

Epilogue

Dear reader – you've made it! You have allowed yourself to be showered with systemic ideas and somehow you got to the end. Perhaps you skipped a lot of the text or, like with a scary detective novel, you started at the end. We don't mind, in our circular world any end isn't really the end, it's just another beginning. Maybe it is the beginning for you to have the courage to put some of what you have learned into practice. Ten minutes for the family may have seemed over-ambitious – it is not! Hopefully you have discovered that 'thinking families', thinking system-ically, is almost always a useful frame when dealing with patients, no matter whether it is just one or five people in the room with you. And you don't even need 10 minutes for it – as we hope we have demonstrated. You have also discovered that the asking of questions is often more useful than the giving of answers. But what will you make of it all? Are you going to use any of it, or will the text of this book just remain a collection of words, with its cover collecting dust? What are the chances of you translating any of the words into action? Please let us know, we are ever so curious.

And if this was not really the end of our book, we would, of course, give you some more seeds for planting. But we won't, because we think that by now you can plant many seeds yourself. So all we authors can do at this stage is to speculate about what stories you might tell us in a year's time. Which ideas and techniques you managed – and which you found utterly useless. And we leave it entirely to you to speculate about how we, the authors, might be affected by what we hear from you. But then, perhaps from that could come another new story, told by you and us.

References

Ackerman, N.W. (1966) *Treating the Troubled Family*. New York: Basic Books.

Altschuler, J. (1997) *Working with Chronic Illness*. Basingstoke and London: Macmillan Press.

Andersen, T. (1987) The reflecting team: dialogue and meta-dialogue in clinical work. *Family Process* **26**: 415–428.

Anderson, C.M. (1983) A psychoeducational program for families of patients with schizophrenia. In: W.-R. McFarlane (ed.) *Family Therapy in Schizophrenia*. New York: Guilford Press.

Anderson, H., Goolishian, H.A. and Windermand, P. (1986) Problem determined systems: toward transformation in family therapy. *Journal of Strategic and Family Therapy* **4**: 1–13.

Asen, E. (1998) On the brink – managing suicidal teenagers. In: P. Sutcliffe, G. Tufnell and U. Cornish (eds) *Working with the Dying and Bereaved*. Basingstoke and London: Macmillan Press.

Asen, E. (2001) Family therapy with ageing families. In: R. Jacoby and C. Oppenheim (eds) *Psychiatry in the Elderly*, 3rd edn. Oxford and New York: Oxford University Press.

Asen, E. and Tomson, P. (1992) *Family Solutions in Family Practice*. Lancaster: Quay Publishing.

Balint, E., Courtenay, M., Elder, A., Hull, S. and Julian, P. (1993) *The Doctor, the Patient and the Group. Balint Revisited*. London: Routledge.

Balint, M. (1957) *The Doctor, His Patient and The Illness*, millennium edition (2000). Edinburgh: Churchill Livingstone.

Bateson, G. (1972) *Steps to an Ecology of Mind: Collected Essays in Anthropology, Psychiatry, Evolution and Epistemology*. London: Chandler.

Bateson, G., Jackson, D., Haley, J. and Weakland, J. (1956) Toward a theory of schizophrenia. *Behavioural Science* **1**: 251–264.

Berg, I.M. (1991) *Family Preservation: A Brief Therapy Workbook*. London: BT Press.

Bing, E. (1970) The conjoint family drawing. *Family Process* **9**: 173–194.

Bloch, D.A. (1987) Family, disease, therapeutic system: the field and the journal. *Family Systems Medicine* **1**: 3.

Bloch, D.A. and Doherty, W.J. (1998) The collaborative family health care coalition. *Families, Systems and Health* **16**: 3–5.

Blount, A. (1998) *Integrated Primary Care: The Future of Medical & Mental Health Collaboration*. New York: W.W. Norton & Company.

Boscolo, L. and Betrando, P. (1996) *Systemic Therapy with Individuals*. London: Karnac Books.

Boscolo, L., Cecchin, G., Hoffman, L. and Penn, P. (1987) *Milan Systemic Family Therapy: Theoretical and Practical Aspects*. New York: Harper & Row.

Bowen, M. (1978) *Family Therapy in Clinical Practice*. New York: Jason Aronson.

Boyd-Franklin, N. (1989) *Black Families in Therapy: A Multisystems Approach*. New York: Guilford Press.

Boyd-Franklin, N. and Franklin, A.J. (1998) African American couples in therapy. In: M. McGoldrick (ed.) *Re-Visioning Family Therapy*. New York and London: Guilford Press.

Burck, C. and Daniel, G. (1995) *Gender and Family Therapy*. London: Karnac Books.

Burns, R.C. and Harvard Kaufman, S. (1970) *Kinetic Family Drawing: An Introduction to Understanding Children through Kinetic Drawings*. New York: Bruner/Mazel.

Byng-Hall, J. (1995) *Rewriting Family Scripts*. New York: Guilford Press.

Carter, E. and McGoldrick, M. (eds) (1989) *The Changing Family Life Cycle*, 2nd edn. Boston, MA: Allyn & Bacon.

Cecchin, G. (1987) Hypothesising, circularity and neutrality revisited: an invitation to curiosity. *Family Process* **26**: 405–413.

Christie-Seely, J. (1984) *Working with Families in Primary Care*. New York: Praeger.

Cole-Kelly, K. (1992) Illness stories and patient care in the family practice context. *Metro Health Medical Center* **24**(1): 45–48.

Cooper, D. (1971) *The Death of the Family*. Harmondsworth: Penguin Books.

Cooperrider, D. (1990) *Appreciative Management and Leadership: The Power of Positive Thought and Action in Organizations*. San Francisco: Jossey-Bass.

Cummings, N.A., Cummings, J.L. *et al.* (1997) *Behavioral Health in Primary Care: A Guide for Clinical Integration*. Madison, CT: Psychosocial Press.

Dallos, R. and Draper, R. (2000) *An Introduction to Family Therapy*. Buckingham and Philadelphia: Open University Press.

de Shazer, S. (1982) *Patterns of Brief Therapy: An Ecosystemic Approach*. New York: Guilford Press.

Doherty, W.J. and Campbell, T.L. (1988) *Families and Health*. Beverly Hills: Sage.

Dowrick, C. (1992) Why do the O'Sheas consult so often? An exploration of complex family illness behaviour. *Social Science Medicine* **34**: 491–497.

D'Zurilla, T.J. (1986) *Problem-solving Therapy: A Social Competence Approach to Clinical Interventions*. New York: Springer.

Elder, A. (1996) Primary care and psychotherapy. *Psychoanalytic Psychotherapy* Suppl. 10.

Elder, A. and Holmes, J. (2002) *Mental Health in Primary Care – A New Approach*. Oxford: Oxford University Press.

Engel, G. (1977) The need for a new medical model: a challenge for biomedicine. *Science* **196**: 129–136.

Engel, G.L. (1980) The clinical application of the biophysical model. *American Journal of Psychiatry* **137**: 535–544.

Fadiman, A. (1997) *The Spirit Catches You and You Fall Down: A Hmong Child, her American Doctors, and the Collision of two Cultures*. New York: The Noonday Press.

Falicov, C. (1998) The cultural meaning of family triangles. In: M. McGoldrick (ed.) *Re-Visioning Family Therapy*. New York and London: Guilford Press.

Falloon, I.R.H. (1988) *Handbook of Behavioural Family Therapy*. New York and London: Guilford Press.

Ferreira, A.J. (1963) Family myths and homeostasis. *Archives of General Psychiatry* **9**: 457–463.

Foucault, M. (1975) *The Archaeology of Knowledge*. London: Tavistock.

Frank, A.W. (1995) *The Wounded Storyteller: Body, Illness and Ethics*. Chicago and London: The University of Chicago Press.

Fredman, G. (1997) *Death Talk: Conversations with Children and Families*. London: Karnac Books.

Geddes, M. and Medway, J. (1977) The symbolic drawing of the family life space. *Family Process* **16**: 219–228.

Goldner, V. (1988) Generation and gender: normative and covert hierarchies. *Family Process* **27**: 17–31.

Goldner, V. (1992) Making room for both/and. *Family Therapy Networker* **16**: 55–61.

Goldner, V., Penn, P., Sheinberg, M. and Walker, G. (1990) Love and violence: gender paradoxes in volatile attachments. *Family Process* **29**: 343–364.

Goolishian, H. and Anderson, H. (1987) Language systems and therapy: an evolving idea. *Psychotherapy* **24**: 529–38.

Greenhalgh, T. and Hurwitz, B. (1998) *Narrative Based Medicine*. London: BMJ Books.

Griffith, J.L. and Griffith, M.E. (1992) Speaking the unspeakable: use of the reflecting position in therapies for somatic symptoms. *Family Systems Medicine* **10**: 41–58.

Haley, J. (1963) *Strategies of Psychotherapy*. New York: Gruner and Stratton.

Haley, J. (1979) *Leaving Home: Therapy for Disturbed Young People*. San Francisco: Jossey-Bass.

Hammond, S.A. (1996) *The Thin Book of Appreciative Inquiry*. Lima, OH: CSS Publishing.

Hardwick, P.J. (1989) Families' medical myths. *Journal of Family Therapy* **11**: 3–27.

Hardy, K.V. and Laszloffy, T.A. (1995) The cultural genogram: key to training culturally competent family therapists. *Journal of Marital and Family Therapy* **21**: 227–237.

Hare-Mustin, R.T. (1991) Sex, lies and headaches: the problem is power. *Journal of Feminist Family Therapy* **3**: 39–61.

Hoffman, L. (2002) *Family Therapy: an Intimate Journey*. New York: W.W.Norton & Co.

Howe, A. (1996) Detecting psychological distress: can general practitioners improve their own performance? *British Journal of General Practice*. **46**: 407–410.

Hurwitz, B. (2000) Narrative and the practice of medicine. *Lancet* **356**: 2086–2089.

Huygen, F.J.A. (1978) *Family Medicine: The Medical Family History of Families*. London: The Royal College of Practitioners.

Jenkins, H. and Asen, K.E. (1992) Family therapy without the family: a framework for systemic practice. *Journal of Family Therapy* **14**: 1–14.

Jones, E. (1993) *Family Systems Therapy: Developments in the Milan-Systemic Therapies*. Chichester: John Wiley & Sons.

Jones, E. and Asen, E. (2000*) Systemic Couple Therapy and Depression*. London and New York: Karnac Books.

Karpman, S., Stewart, I. and Joines, V. (1987) *Transactional Analysis Today*. Lifespace Publications.

Katon, W., Von Korff, M., Lin, E. *et al.* (1990) Distressed high utilisers of medical care, DSM-111-R diagnoses and treatment needs. *General Hospital Psychiatry* **12**: 355–362.

Kleinman, A. (1988) *The Illness Narratives: Suffering, Healing and the Human Condition*. New York: Basic Books.

Kleinman, A. (1995) *Writing at the Margin. Discourse between Anthropology and Medicine*. Berkeley and London: University of California Press.

Kuipers, L., Leff, J. and Lam, D. (1992) *Family Work for Schizophrenia: A Practical Guide*. London: Gaskell.

Laing, R.D. and Esterson, A. (1964) *Sanity, Madness and the Family*. London: Tavistock.

Launer, J. (1996) Toward systemic general practice. *Context* **26**: 42–45.

Launer, J. (2002) *Narrative-based Primary Care – A Practical Guide*. Abingdon: Radcliffe Medical Press.

Leff, J., Kuipers, E., Berkowitz, R., Eberleinfries, R. and Sturgeon, D. (1982) A controlled trial of social intervention in schizophrenic families. *British Journal of Psychiatry* **141**: 121–134.

Majors, R. and Billson, J.M. (1992) *Cool Pose: The Dilemmas of Black Manhood in America*. New York: Lexington Books.

Mason, B. (1993) Towards positions of safe uncertainty. *Human Systems* **4**: 189–200.

Mason, B. (2003) A relational approach to the understanding, treatment and management of chronic pain. Unpublished doctoral thesis. Institute of Family Therapy, London.

Maturana, H. and Varela, F.J. (1980) *Autopoesis and Cognition: The Realization of the Living*. Dordrecht: D. Reidel.

McDaniel, S., Campbell, T. and Seaburn, D. (1990) *Family-oriented Primary Care*. New York: Springer-Verlag.

McGoldrick, M. (1998) A framework for re-visioning family therapy. In: M. McGoldrick (ed.) *Re-Visioning Family Therapy*. New York and London: Guilford Press.

McWhinney, I.R. (1995) Why we need a new clinical method. In: S. Stewart, J. Belle Brown, W.W. Weston, I.R. McWhinney, C.L. McWilliam and T.R. Freeman (eds) *Patient-Centered Medicine: Transforming the Clinical Method*. London: Sage.

Minuchin, S. (1974) *Families and Family Therapy*. London: Tavistock.

Minuchin, S. and Fishman, H.C. (1981) *Family Therapy Techniques*. Cambridge, MA: Harvard University Press.

Morgan, A. (2000) *What is Narrative Therapy?* Adelaide: Dulwich Centre Publications.

Mumford, E., Schlesinger, H.J. *et al.* (1982) The effects of psychological intervention on recovery from surgery and heart attacks: an analysis of the literature. *American Journal of Public Health* **72**: 141–151.

Mynors-Wallis, L.M., Gath, D.H. *et al.* (1995) Randomized controlled trial comparing problem solving treatment with amitriptyline and placebo for major depression in primary care. *British Medical Journal* **310**: 441–445.

Neighbour, R.H. (1987) *The Inner Consultation.* Lancaster: MTP Press.

O'Dowd, T.C. (1988) Five years of heartsink patients in general practice. *British Medical Journal* **297**: 528–530.

Pearce, W.B. and Cronen, V.E. (1980) *Communication, Action and Meaning.* New York: Praeger.

Perelberg, R. and Miller, A. (1990) *Gender and Power in Families.* London: Routledge.

Plsek, P.E. and Greenhalgh, T. (2001) Complexity science: the challenge of complexity in health care. *British Medical Journal* **323**: 625–628.

Plsek, P.E. and Wilson, T. (2001) Complexity science: complexity, leadership, and management in healthcare organisations. *British Medical Journal* **323**: 746–749.

Rolland, J.S. (1987) Towards a psychosocial typology of chronic and life-threatening illness. *Family Process* **26**: 203–221.

Sackett, D.L., Rosenberg, W.M.C., Gray, J.A.M., Haynes, R.B. and Richardson, W.S. (1996) Evidence based medicine: what it is and what it isn't. *British Medical Journal* **312**: 71–72.

Salinsky, J. and Sackin, P. (2000) *What are you Feeling, Doctor? Identifying and Avoiding Defensive Patterns in the Consultation.* Oxford: Radcliffe Medical Press.

Satir, V. (1972) *Peoplemaking.* Palo Alto: Science and Behaviour Books.

Schön, D. (1983) *The Reflective Practitioner.* London: Temple Smith.

Seaburn, D.B., Lorenz, A.D., Gunn, W.B., Gavinski, B.A. and Mauksch, L. (1996) *Models of Collaboration: A Guide for Mental Health Professionals Working with Health Care Practitioners.* New York: Basic Books.

Selvini Palazzoli, M., Boscolo, L., Cecchin, G. and Prata, G. (1978) *Paradox and Counterparadox: A New Model in the Therapy of the Family in Schizophrenic Transaction.* New York: Jason Aronson.

Selvini Palazzoli, M., Boscolo, L., Cecchin, G. and Prata, G. (1980) Hypothesizing-circularity-neutrality; three guidelines for the conductor of the session. *Family Process* **19**: 3–12.

Selvini Palazzoli, M., Cirillo, S., Selvini, M. & Sorrentino, A. (1989) *Family Games.* London: Karnac Books.

Silverman, J., Kurtz, S. and Draper, J. (1998) *Skills for Communicating with Patients.* Abingdon: Radcliffe Medical Press.

Skynner, R. (1976) *One Flesh: Separate Persons. Principles of Family and Marital Therapy.* London: Constable.

Stone, E. (1989) *Black Sheep and Kissing Cousins; How our Family Stories Shape Us.* New York: Penguin.

van Lawick, J. and Groen, M. (1998) *The Spiral of Violence.* Personal Communication.

Von Foerster, H. and Zopf, G.W. (eds) (1962) *Principles of Self-Organization.* New York: Pergamon.

Waldegrave, C. (1998) The challenges of culture to psychology and postmodern thinking. In: M. McGoldrick (ed.) *Re-Visioning Family Therapy.* New York and London: Guilford Press.

Walters, M., Carter, B. and Papp, P. (1988) *The Invisible Web: Gender Patterns in Family Relationships.* New York: Guilford Press.

Watzlawick, P., Jackson, D. and Beavin, J. (1967) *Pragmatics of Human Communication.* New York: W.W. Norton.

Watzlawick, P., Weakland, J. and Fisch, R. (1974) *Change: Principles of Problem Formation and Problem Resolution.* New York: W.W. Norton.

Westhead, J.N. (1985) Frequent attenders in general practice: medical and social characteristics. *Journal of the Royal College of General Practice* **35**: 337–340.

White, M. (1989) *Selected Papers*. Adelaide: Dulwich Centre Publications.

White, M. (1997) *Narratives of Therapists' Lives*. Adelaide: Dulwich Centre Publications.

White, M. and Epston, D. (1990) *Narrative Means to Therapeutic Ends*. New York: W.W. Norton.

Zander, R.S. and Zander, B. (2000) *The Art of Possibility: Transforming Personal and Professional Life*. Cambridge, MA: Harvard Business School Press.

Zigmond, D. (1978) When Balinting is mind-rape. *Psychotherapy*: 1123–1126.

Zimmerman, B., Lindberg, C. and Plsek, P. (2001) *Edgeware: Insights from Complexity Science for Heath Care Leaders*. Irving, TX: VHA.

Index

A-affect (PPRACTICE) 108–9; case vignette
  108–9
addiction-related problems: xiii
adherence *see* compliance, adherence and
  concordance
adolescence 98–9; case vignette 99
advantages of couple work 124–5
ageing: perceptions 101
agenda *see* questioning and reflecting on
  agenda
alliances and coalitions 150
anticipating and rehearsing 153; crisis points
  153
appraisal team: xi
appreciative inquiry 9
approach applicability: xii–xiv; addiction-
  related problems, xiii; children with
  problems, xiii; clinicians, xiv; concordance
  problems, xiii–xiv; family crisis, xiii;
  health promotion work, xiv; multiple
  attenders, xii–xiii; patients with emotional
  problems, xiii; primary care teams, xiv;
  somatically fixated patients, xii
assertive outreach teams 7
assessing, reflecting and connecting 102–22;
  I-illness history 109; C-communication
  109; C-community resources 112; A-affect
  108–9; communication and meta-
  communication 110; culture and gender
  115–16; E-environmental factors 112–13;
  emotions 108; entering political arena
  112; extending hypothesising 114–19;
  family of origin (FOO) group work 118;
  family structures 107; P-presenting
  problem 104; P-problem solving 104–5;
  PPRACTICE 102–13, 122; R-roles, rules
  and responsibilities 105–8; reflection
  113–14; systemic assessment 102–4; T-
  time in life cycle 109–11; time out
  119–21; time out for clinicians 121; time
  to spare 113

Balint, Michael 44; family of origin (FOO)
  group work 118
Bateson,G. 4
becoming a couple 92–5; case vignette 95;
  culture 96
becoming parents 95–6
bio-psycho-social (BPS) 14–15
biomedical model 20–1
blame game 166–8; case vignettes 166–7;
  Drama Triangle 166–8
blame and responsibility 132
both/and positions 165
boundaries 25; disturbances 24
BPS *see* bio-psycho-social
British health system in middle age 186
burn out 179–80

C-communication (PPRACTICE) 109
C-community resources (PPRACTICE) 112;
  Family Circles Method 112
care programme approach (CPA) 143
case conferences 143
categories of crisis 161
central idea: xi–xii; case vignette, xi–xii;
  multiple contexts, xi; stuck situation, xii;
  working with family, xi
chair work 60–3, 133–4
change questions 56
changing work methods 188; case vignette
  188
children with problems: xiii
clinical behaviour 159
clinical governance 7
clinician: as observer or participant 38; stuck,
  bored or burnt out, xiv
CMM *see* coordinated management of
  meaning
collaboration in primary care 185;
  Collaborative Family Health Care
  Coalition 185
collaborative relationship 184–5

communication and meta-communication 110; blamer 110; computer 110; distractor 110; placator 110
complexity: management 7; theory 8
compliance, adherence and concordance 12
computer 8; as consultation member 9; genograms 74
concordance: problems, xiii–xiv, *see also* compliance, adherence and concordance
confidentiality 8, 126, 146, 189
connections between ideas about change 151
consulting to partners 129–30; basic rules 129; case vignette 130
content feedback 50; case vignette 51–2; process feedback 50–2, *see also* feedback
content and process 46
context: definition 1; and family, viii, *see also* organising contexts
continuing to explore 80–1
convening the couple 127–8; dynamics 127; fears 128; violence and risk 128
convening family meetings 143–4
coordinated management of meaning (CMM) 2
coping strategies 166, 168–9, 177; case vignette 179; clinicians 179–80; solution diagram 168–9; tough love 169
corrective scripts 65
couple factor 142
couple work 123–42; advantages 124–5; blame and responsibility 132; consulting to partners 129–30; convening the couple 127–8; couple factor 142; domestic violence 140–2; enactment 135–6; evaluation 136; externalising the relationship 133–4; getting concrete 134–5; health centre poster 125; indications for involving partner 124; joining 132; joining each partner and clarifying issue 131–3; lifestyle changes and health concerns 139–40; limits of couple work 136–7; orienting couple work 130–1; parental history 140; practical issues 123–4; secrets 137–9; ten minutes for couple 137; therapy or consultation 124; three-person consultations 125–7; time out programmes 141; turning individual complaint into couple issue 128–9
CPA *see* care programme approach
crisis 160–2; points 153
Cronen, C. E. 2
cultural considerations 26–7
culture: becoming a couple 96; and gender 115–16; transition points 91

culture of the individual 2–4; consulting behaviours 3; society 2; systemic practice 3–4
curiosity 49; importance 48–50

dance spotting 29, 147
dancing with the family *see* family consultation
DAPHNE 10
data protection 8
default mode 182–5; settings 183
denial 170; integrity protector 170
depression 170–2; case vignettes 171; obesity 171–2
diary 23, 153–4; use 22
disengaged communication patterns 24
domestic violence 140–2; neutrality 141
don't just think families, think context 162
Dowrick, C. 193
Drama Triangle: blame game 166–8
drawing circles 79–80

E-environmental factors (PPRACTICE) 112–13
early crisis intervention teams 7
eating disorders 177–8; anorexia 177; bulimia 178; case vignette 178, *see also* somatisation
emotions 108
empty nest 99–100; case vignette 100
enacting problems 151–2; case vignette 152; soft and tough approaches 152–3
enactment 135–6; interventive questions 135–6
enmeshed families 24, 26
entering political arena 112
evaluation 136
even-handedness 131–2
evolution of systemic work 32–44; Balint and beyond 44; clinician as observer or participant 38; future histories 44; history 32–3; Milan systemic approach 37–8; miracle question 43; noticing and using transference 34; observing, challenging, enacting 36; positive connotation 39; psycho-educational approach 42–4; psychoanalytic family therapy 33; reflecting teams 41; scapegoat practices 33; social constructionist approach 39–40; solution-focused therapy 42; strategic family therapy 36–7; structural approach 33–6; systemic narrative therapy 40–2; tasks 37; transference and you 34
experts by experience 7
exploring: illness 82; relationships 81–2

exploring time 82–8; case vignettes 84–8

extending hypothesising 114–19; case vignette 114–15; hypotheses and interventions 116–19

externalisation of problems 40, 82

externalising questions (chair work) 60–3; case vignettes 61–3

externalising the relationship 133–4; case vignette 134; chair work 133–4

Fadiman, A. 27

familial self 117

family: xi; configuration and life cycle stage 116–17; coping strategies 165; crisis, xiii; dance 27–9, 176; definition 14–15; life cycle 90; members 13; patterns and scripts 64; structures 107; systems model 20–1; within us *see* genograms

family beliefs, myths, scripts 64–6; case vignette 66; corrective scripts 65; family narratives 65–6; replicative scripts 65

Family Circles Method 78–89; C-community resources (PPRACTICE) 112; caveat 88–9; continuing to explore 80–1; drawing circles 79–80; exploring illness 82; exploring relationships 81–2; exploring time 82–8; family circle drawings 88; whole family work 88; working with circles 80; your family circle 89

family consultation 143–9; alliances and coalitions 150; anticipating and rehearsing 153; conclusions 159; connections between ideas about change 151; convening family meetings 143–4; dance spotting 147; enacting problems 151–2; family meeting 144–6; homework tasks 153–4; indirect challenging 156; joining the family 148–9; opening 149–50; paradoxical interventions 157–8; parents stepping out 154–6; reason for family meeting 150; room preparation 148; summing up messages 157; thinking families in severe or chronic illness 144; triadic questioning 150–1; working with families 146–8

family as context: vii–viii ; stuck feeling, viii; vignette, vii–viii

family in crisis 160–80; blame game 166–8; both/and positions 165; burn out 179–80; case vignettes 161–2; categories of crises 161; categories of crisis 161; coping strategies 166, 168–9, 177; crises 160–2; denial 170; depression 170–2; don't just think families – think context 162; drivers 160; eating disorders 177–8; family coping strategies 164; glad game 169–70; pain-full relationships 175; painful stories 174–7; permission 178–9; resilient strategies 172–3; roar the other side of silence 174; sharing the load 180; somatisation 173–4; template for thinking about family crises 162–4; understanding coping strategies 165–6; your crises 161

family in later life 100–1; case vignette 101

family meeting 144–6; barriers 146; case vignette 145; confidentiality 146; invitations 146; power 145–6; Psychiatry for the Elderly 145; risk 146; secrets 146; viability 144–5

family narratives 65–8; case vignette 68; narrative therapy 66

family of origin (FOO) 183–4; Balint, Michael 118; genogram 183–4; group work 118; supervision 183

family styles 25–6; case vignettes 25–6

family as system 23–5; boundary disturbances 24; disengaged communication patterns 24; enmeshed families 24; privacy 24

family transitions 90–101; adolescence 98–9; becoming a couple 92–5; becoming parents 95–6; empty nest 99–100; exercises 97; family in later life 100–1; family life cycle 90; growing children 96–8; life cycle stages 93; perceptions of ageing 101; transition points 91–2; Western family life cycle phases and problems 94

family tree 68–73; genogram 68–9; making connections 72–3; non-verbal feedback 69–72

fat file syndrome: xii

feedback 28, 50; loop 184

FOO *see* family of origin

Foucault, M. 39

fruits: xv 184, *see also* roots, trunk, shoots, fruits, seeds

future histories 44

gender issues 15

general practice 11–12

genograms 64–77, 131, 189; appropriate time 74; case vignettes 66, 68, 74–6; family beliefs, myths, scripts 64–6; family narratives 66–8; family patterns and scripts 64; family tree 68–73; medical myths 67; myths 65; practical considerations 73–4; record keeping 74; seed 67; summary 77; and whole family 75–7 getting concrete 134–5; case vignette 134–5; nodal points 134

glad game 169–70; case vignettes 169–70

growing children 96–8; case vignettes 96–8

headaches for patients and clinicians 11–12; general practice 11–12; patients with emotional problems 11–12; psychological perspective 12

health authorities (HAs) 186

health care systems and change mechanisms 7–8; case vignettes 7–8; systemic practice 7–8; systems theory 7; vocabulary 7; Western health care systems 7

health centre poster 125

health promotion work: xiv

heartsink patients: xii

help questions 55

history of systemic approach 32–3; Bateson, Gregory 32; family therapy 33

homeostasis 25, 106–8; case vignette 107

homework tasks 153–4; case vignette 154; couples 154; diaries 153–4

human resources 7

Huygen, F. J. A. 31

hypotheses 182

hypotheses and interventions 116–19; family configuration and life cycle stage 116–17; presenting problems and cultural patterns 117–19; social situation and symptoms 119; symptom function 119, *see also* extending hypothesising

hypothetical questions 57

I-illness history (PPRACTICE) 109; case vignettes 111

ICE *see* ideas, concerns and expectations

ideas, concerns and expectations (ICE) 182

illness stories 52

indications for involving partner 124

indirect challenging 156; focus 156; neutrality 156

individual: xii; self 117, *see also* culture of the individual

information technology 8

integrated practice 4–5

interactional approach: viii

interventive, non-blaming approaches 20–1; biomedical model 20–1; family systems model 20–1

interventive questions: enactment 135–6

job descriptions: team relationship 187–8

joining 132, 159

joining each partner and clarifying issue 131–3; even-handedness 131–2; genogram 131; mirroring 131–3; non-verbal clues 131; stuckness 133

joining the family 148–9; engagement 149; introduction 149

knowledge tree: xv; fruits, xv; roots, xv; seeds, xv; shoots, xv

Laing, R. D.: blame and responsibility 132

learning organisations 7

life cycle stages 93

lifestyle changes and health concerns 139–40

limits of couple work 136–7; concrete issues 136; focus 136

linear thinking limits 6, *see also* positivism and linear causality

living context 1

load *see* sharing the load

McWhinney, I. R. 6

medical myths 67

mental health subgroup: xi

Milan systemic approach 37–8; parents stepping out 155

miracle question 43, 58–60; case vignettes 58–60

miracle seeds working on organisational system 189

mirroring 131–3

multi-person meetings 143

multiple attenders: xii-xiii

multiple contexts: xi

multiple perspectives 19

muscle memory level 182

myths 65

narrative therapy 66

narrative-based primary care practitioners 40

narratives *see* patients' stories

National Health Service 186

network meetings 143

non-verbal clues 131

non-verbal feedback 69–72

obesity: depression 171–2

observing, challenging, enacting 36

opening 149–50

organising contexts: context definition 1; living context 1; person context 1; reframing 2; for team and patients 1–2; ten-minute consultation 1

orientation 159

orienting couple work 130–1; relationship problem 131
outputs 7

P-presenting problem (PPRACTICE) 104; chair work 104
P-problem solving (PPRACTICE) 104–5
pain perspectives 5
pain-full relationships 175
painful stories 174–7; case vignettes 175–7; chronic pain 174–7
paper on systemic ideas 31
paradoxical interventions 157–8; case vignette 158
parental history 140
parents stepping out 154–6; Milan School of family therapy 155
partners in service design 7
partnerships 7
Patient Participation groups 186
patients 11; with emotional problems, xiii 11–12; stories 17–19, *see also* service user
Pearce, W.B. 2
performance management 7
permission 178–9
person context 1
person, family and others 13–14; case vignettes 14
positive connotation 39, *see also* reframing
positivism and linear causality 5–6; case vignette 6
power of questions 52–3
PPRACTICE 102–4, 189; P-presenting problem 104; P-problem solving 104–5; R-roles, rules, responsibilities 105–8; A-affect 108–9; C-communication 109; T-time in life cycle 109; I-illness history 109–11; C-community resources 112; E-environmental factors 112–13; nine dimensions 103
practical issues: in couple work 123–4
practice system 29; case vignette 29; spotting 31
practice systems: and family systems 29–31
practice team: xi
PREP plan 183
presenting problems and cultural patterns 117–19; familial self 117; individual self 117; matriarchal families 117–18
primary care: collaboratives 7; population 9
primary care changes 8–10; computer 8; confidentiality 8; DAPHNE 10; data protection 8; information technology 8; primary care population 9; units of delivery 8

primary care clinician: key ingredients, xiv–xv; relationships, xi
primary case team: xi
privacy 24
problem-determined system 39
problem/symptom questions 54
psycho-educational approach 42–4; Meriden project 44
psychoanalytic family therapy 33; containing stance 33; counter-transference 33
psychological perspective 12

question types 52–7; reflexive and circular question examples 54–7
questioning and reflecting on agenda 45–63; content feedback 50; content and process 46; curiosity 49; externalising questions (chair work) 60–3; feedback 50; illness stories 52; importance of curiosity 48–50; miracle question 58–60; power of questions 52–3; practice suggestion 55; practice task 59, 63; question types 52–7; questioning the symptom: reflective practice 47; questioning the symptom 46–8; systemic approach 45–6; three questions for you 63
questioning the symptom 46–8, 191; case vignette 48; reflective practice 47

R-roles, rules and responsibilities (PPRACTICE) 105–8; case vignette 106; Dr Homeostat 106–8
reason for family meeting 150
receptionist as systemic practitioner 30
record keeping 74
reflecting teams 41
reflection 113–14
reflexive and circular question examples: change questions 56; help questions 55; hypothetical questions 57; problem/symptom questions 54; relationship questions 56; solution-focused questions 54–5; wild questions 57
reframing 2, 159, *see also* positive connotation
relationship: of individuals, viii; questions 56
relationship lens 12–13; case vignettes 12–13; family members 13
replicative scripts 65
resilient strategies 172–3; case vignettes 172–3
ripple effect: xii
roar the other side of silence 174
room preparation: family meeting 148

roots: xv, *see also* roots, trunk, shoots, fruits, seeds
roots, trunk, shoots, fruits, seeds 181–91; British health system in middle age 186; changing work methods 188; collaboration in primary care 185; collaborative relationship 184–5; default mode settings 183; feedback loop 184; miracle seeds working on organisational system 189; systemic practice 181–2; systemic practitioners involvement 188–90; team relationship 185–8; toolbox 181; work mode 182–3; working on the family of origin (FOO) 183–4
Royal College of General Practitioners: ICE 182

scapegoat practices 33
secrets 137–9; case vignette 138; pacing 138
seeds: xv 184, *see also* roots, trunk, shoots, fruits, seeds
service user 11
sharing the load 180
shoots: xv, *see also* roots, trunk, shoots, fruits, seeds
social constructionist approach 39–40; Foucault, M. 39; narrative-based primary care practitioners 40; problem-determined system 39
social situation and symptoms 119
solution-focused: questions 54–5; therapy 42
somatisation: xii 173–4; case vignettes 173–4
split bodies and minds 4–5; case vignette 5; integrated practice 4–5
stakeholders 7
storytellers 19
strategic family therapy 36–7
stress: family 91–2
structural approach 33–6; case vignettes 35–6
stuck: feeling, viii; situation, xii; stuckness 133
summing up messages 157; praise 157
supervision 189–90
symptom: focus 21–3; function 21, 119
symptoms 19–20; family dimension 19
system 4; stability *see* homeostasis
systemic approach 11–31, 45–6, 191; bio-psycho-social (BPS) 14–15; boundaries 25; compliance, adherence and concordance 12; cultural considerations 26–7; dance spotting 29; diary 23; diary use 22; family 14–15; family dance 27–9; family styles 25–6; family as system 23–5; feedback 28; gender issues 15; headaches for patients and clinicians 11–12;

homeostasis 25; interventive, non-blaming approaches 20–1; multiple perspectives 19; paper on systemic ideas 31; patients' stories 17–19; person, family and others 13–14; practice system 29; practice system spotting 31; practice systems and family systems 29–31; receptionist as systemic practitioner 30; relationship lens 12–13; storytellers 19; symptom focus 21–3; symptom function 21; symptoms 19–20; systemic headaches 11–12; systemic zoom lens 16–17; zoom lens or wide-angle lens 17, *see also* evolution of systemic work
systemic headaches 11–12
systemic narrative therapy 40–2; case vignettes 41–2; externalisation of problems 40; reflecting team 40
systemic practice 1–10, 181–2; appreciative inquiry 9; case vignettes 10; complexity theory 8; computer as consultation member 9; coordinated management of meaning (CMM) 2; culture of the individual 2–4; health care systems and change mechanisms 7–8; linear thinking limits 6; organising contexts for team and patients 1–2; pain perspectives 5; positivism and linear causality 5–6; primary care changes 8–10; split bodies and minds 4–5; system 4, *see also* evolution of systemic work
systemic practitioners involvement 188–90; case vignettes 189–90; supervision 189–90
systemic work in primary care: viii–xi; case vignettes, ix–x; context and family, viii; interactional approach, viii; primary care clinician relationships, xi; relationships of individuals, viii, *see also* evolution of systemic work
systemic zoom lens 16–17; case vignette 16; thinking families 16
systems theory: xii 7

T-time in life cycle (PPRACTICE) 109–11
tapestry of family life 162–3
tasks 37
team relationship 185–8; case vignette 187; job descriptions 187–8; understanding colleagues 185–8
template for thinking about family crises 162–4; case vignettes 163–4; tapestry of family life 162–3
ten-minute consultation 1, 191; for couple 137
therapy or consultation 124

thinking families: xiii 16, 191; in severe or chronic illness 144

three questions for you 63

three-person consultations 125–7; bias 126; case vignette 127; confidentiality 126; couple war 126

time out 119–21; case vignette 120–1; for clinicians 121; programmes 141

time to spare 113

toolbox 181

total quality management 7

transference: noticing and using 34; and you 34

transition points 91–2; case vignettes 92; culture 91, *see also* family transitions

triadic questioning 150–1

trunk: xv, *see also* roots, trunk, shoots, fruits, seeds

turning individual complaint into couple issue 128–9; case vignette 129

understanding coping strategies 165–6

units of delivery 8

Western family life cycle phases 94

whole systems working 7

wild questions 57

work mode 182–3; default mode 182–3; hypotheses 182; ideas, concerns and expectations (ICE) 182; muscle memory level 182; PREP plan 183

working with circles 80

working with families 146–8; consultation as dance 147; reason for meeting 148

your crises 161

your family circle 89

zoom lens or wide-angle lens 17

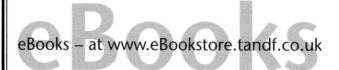